WOMEN'S HEALTH ADVOCACY

Women's Health Advocacy brings together academic studies and personal narratives to demonstrate how women use a variety of arguments, forms of writing, and communication strategies to effect change in a health system that is not only often difficult to participate in, but which can be actively harmful. It explicates the concept of rhetorical ingenuity—the creation of rhetorical means for specific and technical, yet extremely personal, situations. At a time when women's health concerns are at the center of national debate, this rhetorical ingenuity provides means for women to uncover latent sources of oppression in women's health and medicine and to influence matters of research, funding, policy, and everyday access to healthcare in the face of exclusion and disenfranchisement. This accessible collection will be inspiring reading for academics and students in health communication, medical humanities, and women's studies, as well as for activists, patients, and professionals.

Jamie White-Farnham is Associate Professor and Writing Coordinator at the University of Wisconsin-Superior.

Bryna Siegel Finer is Associate Professor and the Director of Writing Across the Curriculum at Indiana University of Pennsylvania.

Cathryn Molloy is Associate Professor and Director of Undergraduate Studies in James Madison University's School of Writing, Rhetoric and Technical Communication.

WOMEN'S HEALTH ADVOCACY

Rhetorical Ingenuity for the 21st Century

Edited by Jamie White-Farnham, Bryna Siegel Finer, and Cathryn Molloy

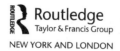

Routledge
Taylor & Francis Group

NEW YORK AND LONDON

First published 2020
by Routledge
52 Vanderbilt Avenue, New York, NY 10017

and by Routledge
2 Park Square, Milton Park, Abingdon, Oxon OX14 4RN

Routledge is an imprint of the Taylor & Francis Group, an informa business

© 2020 Taylor & Francis

The right of the Jamie White-Farnham, Bryna Siegel Finer, and Cathryn Molloy to be identified as the authors of the editorial material, and of the authors for their individual chapters, has been asserted in accordance with sections 77 and 78 of the Copyright, Designs and Patents Act 1988.

Library of Congress Cataloging-in-Publication Data
Names: White-Farnham, Jamie, editor. | Finer, Bryna Siegel, editor. | Molloy, Cathryn, editor.
Title: Women's health advocacy : rhetorical ingenuity for the 21st century / edited by Jamie White-Farnham, Bryna Siegel Finer, Cathryn Molloy.
Description: First edition. | New York, NY : Routledge, 2019. | Includes bibliographic references.
Identifiers: LCCN 2019013988| ISBN 9780367192242 (hardback) | ISBN 9780367192259 (pbk.) | ISBN 9780429201165 (ebook)
Subjects: LCSH: Women patients--Communication. | Communication in medicine. | Patient advocacy. | Women patients--Social conditions--21st century. | Women's health services--Social aspects. | Rhetoric--Social aspects.
Classification: LCC RA564.85 .W6858 2019 | DDC 613/.04244--dc23
LC record available at https://lccn.loc.gov/2019013988

ISBN: 978-0-367-19224-2 (hbk)
ISBN: 978-0-367-19225-9 (pbk)
ISBN: 978-0-429-20116-5 (ebk)

Typeset in Bembo
by Taylor & Francis Books

CONTENTS

FIGURES

ACKNOWLEDGMENTS

Creating an edited collection takes the hard work, collaboration, and the patience of many people. We are indebted to the following:

Jamie White-Farnham would like to thank the faculty and staff of the Writing Program at UW-Superior. The collegiality of this group is beyond compare; thank you. She would also like to thank April Cabral, a WB sister since the age of 4, who has been more than generous with her precious time during this project.

Bryna Siegel Finer would like to thank Sandi Sirotowitz for always being the family healthcare advocate; her parents, Marcia and Howard Siegel for always supporting her writing; and Robin Karlin and the local Pittsburgh and national FORCE community for their inspirational BRCActivism.

Cathryn Molloy would like to thank the faculty and staff at JMU's school of WRTC; her mentors, including Traci Zimmerman, Lisa Melonçon, Blake Scott, Fred Reynolds, Nedra Reynolds, Libby Miles, Kim Hensley-Owens, Ann Green, Bob Schwegler, and Jeremiah Dyehouse; her parents and sisters: Ed, Linda, Irene, Missy, Mary, and Annie Molloy.

We are each "momfessors" with families who support us 100% when our academic interests, passions, and projects spill over onto the soccer sideline and school pick-up line. Each of our husbands and our children, who range in age from 1 to 16 years old, help make time and space for our work when necessary, including vacating houses with children in tow. We thank them all—Steve, Ruby, and Claire Farnham; David and Theo Finer; and Jim and Lucas Raisch. And welcome to the fold, little Mateo Molloy Raisch, who was born during the process of editing this book.

We thank our anonymous reviewers, scholars in the rhetoric of health and medicine, who challenged our assumptions and points of view, strengthening the collection as a whole. We are also grateful to everyone at Routledge who supported this book and its production. Ahmed Mostafa's eye for detail was invaluable to us.

This edited collection in particular required some additional love and care along the way, not only because of the heart-rending topic of this book, but also because the women who made and contributed to it are the people about and for whom we write. Above all, we thank our lay and scholarly contributors, many of whom share the most personal and difficult aspects of their lives because both they, and we, hope it will help others. We are confident it will.

ACRONYM KEY

Many acronyms are used frequently throughout this collection to refer to publications, organizations, companies, medicines, diseases, tests, treatment methods, devices, common medical phrases, and laws—all central elements in the discussion of women's health. Rather than name and explain them repeatedly, they are collected and spelled out here to aid in the reader's understanding and experience.

AAFP	American Association of Family Physicians
AAN!	AIDS Action Now!
AAP	American Association of Pediatrics
AAHP	AIDS Activist History Project
ABOUT	American BRCA★ Outcomes and Utilization of Testing Network
ACA	Affordable Care Act★★
ACIP	Advisory Committee of Immunity Practices
ACOG	American College of Obstetrics and Gynecology
AIDS	Acquired Immune Deficiency Syndrome
AMA	Against medical advice
BFHI	Baby Friendly Hospital Initiative
BFUSA	Baby Friendly United States of America
BLyS	B-lymphocyte stimulator
★BRCA	BReast CAncer gene 1 or 2
CAM	Complementary and Alternative Medicines
CDC	Center for Disease Control and Prevention
DHHS	US Department of Health and Human Services
DTP	Diphtheria, tetanus, and pertussis vaccine for babies
FAM	Fertility Awareness Method

FCM	Feminist Communitarian Model
FDA	Food and Drug Administration
FORCE	Facing Our Risk of Cancer Empowered
GSK	Glaxo-Smith-Kline
HIV	Human Immunodeficiency Virus
HBC	Hormonal Birth Control
HBOC	Hereditary Breast and Ovarian Cancer
HMO	Health Maintenance Organization
HPV	Human Papillomavirus
IUD	Intrauterine device
IRB	Institutional Review Board
ITP	Idiopathic thrombocytopenic purpura
JAMA	*Journal of the American Medical Association*
LGBT	Lesbian, Gay, Bisexual, Transgender community (see also LGBTQIA+)
LGBTQIA+	Lesbian, Gay, Bisexual, Transgender, Queer/Questioning, Intersex, Asexual, Plus (with the "plus" to be inclusive to anyone else who may wish to identify themselves as a member of this community under any additional term or terms)
MGT	Muted Group Theory
MPH	Master's degree in Public Health
MH	Medical Humanities
MS	Multiple Sclerosis
NEJM	*New England Journal of Medicine*
NIH	National Institute of Health
NSAID	Non-steroidal anti-inflammatory drugs
NSGC	National Society of Genetic Counseling
OBGYN	Obstetrician/Gynecologist
OBOS	*Our Bodies, Ourselves*
OWH	Office of Women's Health
PCORI	Patient-Centered Outcomes Research Institute
PCOS	Polycystic Ovary Syndrome
PCP	Primary care physician
PMS	Premenstrual Syndrome
★★PPACA	Patient Protection Affordable Care Act, most commonly referred to as ACA
PT	Physical Therapy
RCT	Random Controlled Trial
RHM	Rhetoric of Health and Medicine
SLE	Systemic Lupus Erythematosus
STI	Sexually Transmitted Infection
TCOYF	*Take Control of Your Fertility*, both the title of a book and a contraceptive method

Tdap	Tetanus, diphtheria, and pertussis booster vaccine for adults
WHO	World Health Organization
UNICEF	United Nations International Children's Emergency Fund
UK	United Kingdom
US	United States

INTRODUCTION

Jamie White-Farnham and Cathryn Molloy

"The best doctors are not intimidated by knowledgeable patients."

Donna Laux, this volume

At a time when women's health concerns are at the center of national debate, women strive to influence matters of research, funding, policy, and everyday access to healthcare. Public examples include Angelina Jolie's announcements of her prophylactic mastectomy and oophorectomy in *The New York Times* as well as Lady Gaga's recent announcement of her fibromyalgia diagnosis, which she shared on social media and in an HBO documentary (Fallon, 2017). We take these personal, yet public rhetorical acts as the type that constitute health activism, or "how the discourses of health and bodily well-being [circulate] among different social movement sectors and [create] grounds for coalition and conflict" (Loyd, 2014).

In 2019, discourses around women's health and bodily well-being are rife with conflict; elaborate legal, corporate, and activist organizations support, provide, govern, require, and often limit women's knowledge, power, and participation in their own health and healthcare. A constant stream of commentary from politicians, government officials, and media pundits analyzes and scrutinizes women and their health choices. Rather than critique the unfair and/or limiting structures in place regarding women's education, access, and options, these comments often over-simplify the complex, rhetorically-rich contexts of health choices, often focusing their attention on the women as pathetic victims, righteous feminists, or worse. In one compelling example, McMillan's chapter in this volume (Chapter 15) points to Rush Limbaugh's slut-shaming of Sandra Fluke—a law student who had the audacity to ask in public for the US government to pay for birth control.

In such a context, the writers and participants whose situations and problems are represented in this volume report that they are unheard, excluded, and disenfranchised. They express discontent with the low level (and sometimes absence) of rhetorical and material control they have over their own bodies. It is no coincidence, given the thrust of arguments against women's health rights heard from Washington.

However, the evidence in the studies herein demonstrates that women do not always accept such treatment. Rather, the research participants, advocates, and activists in this book use surprising and perhaps sobering rhetorical strategies to interrupt, subvert, and affect change in health and healthcare arenas. These practices not only resist threats to women's agency regarding their own health, but they also expand our understanding of rhetorical activism in health and healthcare. Specifically, the writing, arguments, and communication strategies these women rhetors and activists use constitute what we are calling **rhetorical ingenuity—the practice of creating one's own rhetorical means in highly charged, often technical, yet extremely personal, rhetorical situations**. We qualify rhetorical ingenuity as distinct from Aristotelian "available means" of persuasion, which typically necessitate the process of inventing arguments, arranging evidence, and considering counter-arguments. The distinction is necessary because, in the many discourses of healthcare, there is no template, no model, no "rhetoric" for how to gain what patients and activists often say they cannot get from the medical establishment: support, information, other people's narratives, options outside mainstream medical advice, even certain products to bring relief. Still, rhetorical ingenuity involves uncovering latent sources of oppression in women's health and medicine and employing tactics that successful women's health advocates use to push for the care they want for themselves and for other women—all goals that align with RHM.

For instance, our contributor Qadri began her online platform to support patients with Lupus because literally nothing else like her site existed online. In Chapters 3 and 4, McKinley and Pengilly respectively explain how women with PCOS and Lupus seek and share information on online patient forums when medical authorities can't provide them with relief. These women work, sometimes in quite modest and unnoticeable ways, to expose inequities with an eye toward eliminating barriers and rectifying disenfranchising practices. We assert that these rhetors and activists are not only drawing on available means for persuasion, but are also forging ahead with inventive uses of language to affect particular and urgent material changes on behalf of their own and others' health and lives. They also recognize the need to play the "long game" in terms of women's health activism.

Joining the efforts to catalog and understand the ways that such writing and rhetoric are deployed within the context of women's health activism, this collection has two main goals:

1.   to critique the institutional and public discourses that represent, position, or otherwise control women's experiences in healthcare; and

2. to enumerate and make available to a wider audience of patients, advocates, and activists the discourses women use to act and advocate on behalf of their own and others' health and healthcare.

Writing Women, Women('s) Writing

Studies in RHM have focused on the ways that language is used within the medical industrial complex to both limit and afford power to individuals; often documents, policies, and discourses have been found to sublimate and even exclude certain patients. For instance, Emmons (2010) examines the sexist persuasive tactics used in antidepressant advertisements; Jensen (2010) offers critical analysis of early sex education exigencies, actors, and texts; and Keränen (2010) examines the relationship between the public characterization of a physician-researcher and the content and outcome of biomedical research. Writing on women's health in particular, Wells's (2010) *Our Bodies, Ourselves and the Work of Writing* uses archival and interview data to analyze how several editions of *OBOS* and the collective of women responsible for its inception and publication were able to alter everyday women's views of their bodies in relation to biomedicine.

Following suit, our first goal is to present analyses of certain discourses and texts that shape practices and patients. Typically, the findings of such analyses reveal telling gaps, loopholes and catch-22s that women are subject to and which sometimes afford space for resistance. For example, in Chapter 13, Bivens, Cole, and Koerber analyze the discourses surrounding hormonal birth control, which have for a century narrowed women's understanding of how their bodies work; they also highlight two counter-discourses of birth control as alternative means for women who would resist the hegemony of hormonal birth control. In Chapter 6, Whitney offers an analysis of the well-woman exam, arguing that it is rooted in a traditional conception of normative bodies—mainly white women's bodies—that exclude "non-normal" bodies and echo past medical injustices and violence toward women of color. Likewise, DeTora and Malkowski, in Chapter 9, explore competing discourses of safety and danger in maternal vaccinations.

The realities examined as part of our first goal make it clear why women in so many health contexts find themselves compelled to interrupt, resist, or subvert healthcare systems and providers. We, therefore, turn to the second goal of this volume and the counterpart of the analytical approach to the rhetoric of health and medicine—the necessarily creative ways in which women/patients/activists have used their rhetorical ingenuity to speak truth to power or help change conditions, practices, and policies.

Scholarship of the latter type include Molloy's (2015) findings that participants with mental illness in outpatient mental health spaces developed "recuperative ethos" in order to gain the attention and trust of their providers. Similarly, Siegel Finer's (2016) study examined how previvors used blogging to support and inform newly diagnosed community members about their rights before the 2013

Supreme Court decision to overturn Myriad Genetics' patent on the BRCA genes. Further, Gouge's (2010) and Segal's (2008) work on noncompliance call attention to the affordances and limitations of discursive reworkings of common health and medical terminology, and Holladay's (2017) study offers an account of how those with mental disabilities interpret and manipulate medical terminology in online discussions as a way to wrest control away from the medical establishment.

Examples of this type of research include Tadros' interviews with women runners in Chapter 10, who resist doctors' male-centric narratives for their recovery. Additionally, in Chapter 15, interviews with Dean's participants resulted in a four-part model of advocacy for previvors. Cabral similarly challenged medical authorities by demanding a mammogram after finding a breast lump, even when her OBGYN said she did not immediately need one. These contributions are just a few examples of the progressive forms that this type of research can take. We suggest that the growing number of studies such as these have helped to define RHM as necessarily activist. In other words, there is no rhetoric of health and medicine without an imperative to improve conditions. While, of course, our foundational rhetorical theories are grounded in the "truth and justice" of interest to Aristotle, RHM is directed more urgently at language takeaways. It is a project to understand and wield rhetoric not only on behalf of a community with aims for future good, but more stridently for people living and dying who need—and create—resources to improve their conditions, their treatments, and their lives now.

Section Summaries

When we take stock of the rhetorical practices emerging from the research studies featured in this collection, we see three main roles in which women operate rhetorically: Self, Patient, and Activist. In real life, these roles converge and overlap, so we do not take them as fixed, immutable categories. Nevertheless, readers will encounter three main sections organized this way. The studies feature a mix of methodologies, generally aligned with the two purposes of the book: studies of published and/or public texts, as well as studies of informal language use of everyday writers and rhetors.

Rhetoric of the Self

With a focus on individual rhetorical action, this section includes chapters that report on women's self-sponsored writing, such as expressivist writing, writing-to-heal, or writing for educational reasons. Generally speaking, this section is devoted to the creativity of women responding to the circumstances of their health. Writers in this section unpack their own experiences with breast biopsies, athletic injury, cancer, MS, PCOS, and Lupus. Collectively, their chapters make it clear that women's private health stories serve advocacy agendas in circuitous and even fraught ways.

Rhetoric of/and the Patient

This section examines the rhetorical, legal, corporate, and activist systems in which patients participate or struggle in terms of their health. Chapters in this section exemplify the (mis)representations of women within discourses that characterize and create systems and organizations. For example, Gilson, in Chapter 11, analyzes the usability of breastfeeding guidelines to explore how varied users must be considered essential contributors to the process of developing such wide-scale policies. In Chapter 8, Fitzgerald examines HPV advertisements as examples of the gendered nature of discourses of responsibility in health and medical decision-making. This section includes accounts of women who have been unexpectedly ushered into their new lives as public advocates following surprising and daunting diagnoses; the contributors share the sources and consequences of inaccurate health and medical information as that information enters into public opinion.

Rhetorics of Activists

With a focus on public writing and rhetoric, this section includes chapters about the rhetorical movements and arguments made by and on behalf of women in terms of their own health and healthcare. In Chapter 15, for example, McMillan argues that fast arguments in the service of feminism can undermine the bigger picture of equality. That is, McMillan shares how *kairotic* women's health activism does not always align with the goals of long-term, intersectional feminist health and medical goals.

Importantly, chapters in all three sections offer explicit recommendations and/or takeaways for women, patients, and activists who'd like to intervene in their own health and medical realities. These ideas for interventions, we have learned, are not always what an empowered feminist might expect. Some involve strategic compliance or cooperation with authorities in small instances to gain footing for bigger problems (such as in Dean, Chapter 15 and Rysdam, Chapter 7). Some involve adopting a moderate balance between the establishment and what might be seen as "fringey" alternatives (such as Pengilly, Chapter 4) since completely shunning established practices does not always lead to better health outcomes. Some exemplify the maddening ways in which women are written into systems and the rhetorical ways they struggle and only sometimes succeed in using their voices (see Hensley Owens in Chapter 1 and Rysdam in Chapter 7, where both writers describe such struggles). Finally, some involve waiting. Wallace, in Chapter 2, writes about the available discourses of illness before the internet age. She did not write her health narrative for many years, unable to find her voice until wider web authoring practices gave her an audience and a community.

Of course, there are also instances of more obvious and public actions and assertions. Novotny & DeHertogh in Chapter 5, for example, explore their experiences with infertility to suggest the benefits of self-disclosure as activism. Novotny's mock announcement of her "empty womb" helps wider publics appreciate the invisibility that women who have experienced infertility often feel. Klostermann, in Chapter 5, offers archival evidence of the necessarily "loud" methods of women's AIDS activism in Toronto in the 1980s and 1990s; such in-your-face activism was needed to counter the erroneous public perception at the time that only gay men got AIDs.

Expanding Epistemologies and Rhetorics

In addition to academically-framed arguments, this book holds a "third space" that expands the epistemological givens of RHM and the varieties of rhetorical forms the reader will encounter. Specifically, we have invited three non-academic women's health activists to share their knowledge, thoughts, and perspectives on the subject of their rhetorical efforts, including public speaking, fundraising, and social media influence.

Our main reason for doing so is to offer epistemological balance to our understanding of the language used by women/patients/activists. We value the mainstream RHM community and its norms of scholarly writing highly, from logical reasoning to citation practices. However, we are also sensitive to the fact that the research practices of an academic discipline can exclude people who could otherwise reasonably participate in knowledge-making, including the very women whose rhetoric we study.

Therefore, we have invited and are grateful for the presence of writing by women whose writing and rhetoric are crucial to their immediate health contexts and to the larger project of women's health activism. This inclusion amounts to three narrative essays placed throughout this book. Importantly, these contributions are not in academic prose, nor are they researched in the traditional sense. They are solicited essays by women of our acquaintance through activist circles. The women, Donna Laux, Janeen Qadri, and April Cabral, share everyday acts of advocacy that are user-friendly and expedient.

Hope for 2020 and Beyond

In 2008, Heifferon and Brown edited what was arguably the first RHM collection, *The Rhetoric of Healthcare: Essays Toward a New Disciplinary Inquiry*. It featured a study of nursing students, an analysis of the prognosis as genre, an argument for clinical tests as rhetorical process, a case study of the creation of an Occupational Therapy doctorate and its identity-formation, and an argument for medical videos as "composition." Their work foregrounded the "life and death rhetoric" that characterized inquiry in the area (p. 2); it sought to build a corpus for and delineate the content of RHM. Also in 2008, Segal published the highly influential *Health and the Rhetoric of Medicine* in which she described the what, why, and how of studying health and medicine rhetorically and then demonstrated the value of such a theoretical framework via rhetorical inquiries into, for example, hypochondria, death and dying, and patient noncompliance. Of course, since then, the growth of the field is also evidenced by the many excellence monographs and articles cited herein, as well as Lisa Melonçon and Blake Scott's creation of the dynamic new journal, *Rhetoric of Health and Medicine* in 2018.

Initially, we imagined this project would make a timely update to, or pay homage to, Heifferon and Brown (2008), a way to show the advances and changes of the past decade on such studies with a focus on women. We were excited by the variety of research studies in the field—a feature that Melonçon and Scott (2018) identify as a hallmark of RHM. At the same time, we remain conflicted about the number of illnesses and conditions around which women are misrepresented, or poorly informed, misinformed, or limited in their options. The 15 chapters in this book represent research, commentary, and insights into women/patients/activists of an alarming number of illnesses or conditions around which women continue to need and use rhetorical ingenuity, and the tactics herein must be multiplied in coming years. This work has to continue. In some moments, we are indignant that this is the state of modern medicine: when black women have the highest cervical cancer mortality rate (see Chapter 6); when female runners and AIDs patients are treated as small men (see Chapters 10 and 14); and when the *doxa* of hormonal birth control goes unquestioned (Chapter 13).

The 21st century has brought challenges to conditions and attitudes about women's rights to health and safety that are a shock to us, each of us having been born after *Roe v. Wade* and Title IX. Those feminist triumphs, we thought, were our birthright—although as cisgender, heterosexual white women committed to intersectional feminism, we understand that such rights have always been precarious and even callously disregarded for our peers of color, of lower socio-economic status, our LGBTQIA+ peers and those who are disabled. We are especially sensitive to the fact that our transwomen peers are often invisible in conversations on women's health and healthcare. We know that this work only begins to skim the surface of deeply troubling issues that need much more attention. The research in this collection provides specific examples of who and how these retrograde attitudes and policies hurt.

On the other hand, as feminists and rhetoricians, we are encouraged by the groundswell of rhetorical ingenuity this volume represents. It demonstrates the resolve of women who create change for themselves and others. To that end, *Women's Health Advocacy* does not pinkwash or use easy platitudes; it doubles down on the reality of the health and healthcare conditions of women in the early 21st century, exposing injustices and sharing with others not only the available, but the often-ingenious means of direct action to improve conditions. We join (and call on) other rhetoricians, patients, and advocates who do the same.

References

Aristotle. (2004). *Aristotle's Rhetoric*. W. Rhys Roberts (Trans.). Mineola, NY: Dover.

Emmons, K. (2010). *Black dogs and blue words: Depression and gender in the age of self-care.* New Brunswick, NJ: Rutgers University Press.

Fallon, N. (2017). "Fibromyalgia: The pain behind Lady Gaga's poker face." *The Guardian.* Retrieved from www.theguardian.com/science/sifting-the-evidence/2017/oct/02/fibromyalgia-the-pain-behind-lady-gagas-poker-face

Gouge, C.C. (2010). "Health humanities baccalaureate programs and the rhetoric of health and medicine." *Technical Communication Quarterly*, 27(1), 21–32.

Heifferon, B., & Brown, S.C., Eds. (2008). *Rhetoric of healthcare: Essays toward a new disciplinary inquiry.* New York: Hampton Press.

Holladay, A. (2017). "Classified conversations: Psychiatry and tactical technical communication in online space." *Technical Communication Quarterly*, 26(1), 8–24.

Jensen, R.E. (2010). *Dirty words: The rhetoric of public sex education, 1870–1924.* Urbana, IL: University of Illinois.

Keränen, L. (2010). *Scientific characters: Rhetoric, politics, and trust in breast cancer research.* Tuscaloosa, AL: University of Alabama Press.

Loyd, J.M. (2014). *Health rights are civil rights: Peace and justice activism in Los Angeles, 1963–1978.* Minneapolis, MN: University of Minnesota Press.

Melonçon, L., & Scott, J.B. (2018). *Methodologies for the rhetoric of health and medicine.* New York: Routledge.

Molloy, C. (2015). "Recuperative ethos and agile epistemologies: Toward a vernacular engagement with mental illness ontologies." *Rhetoric Society Quarterly*, 45(2), 138–163.

Segal, J.Z. (2008). *Heath and the Rhetoric of Medicine.* Carbondale, IL: Southern Illinois University Press.

Siegel Finer, B. (2016). "The rhetoric of previving: Blogging the breast cancer gene." *Rhetoric Review*, 35(2), 176–188.

Wells, S. (2010). *Our bodies ourselves and the work of writing.* Redwood City, CA: Stanford University Press.

SECTION 1
Rhetorics of Self

With a focus on individual rhetorical action, this section includes chapters that report on women's self-sponsored writing, such as expressivist writing, writing-to-heal, or writing for educative practices. Generally speaking, this section is devoted to the creativity of women responding to the circumstances of their health.

ADVOCATE

Donna Laux

My first period lasted 14 days. That might have been a clue that all was not well reproductively. By 15, I was enduring extreme periods to the point of passing out in school from iron deficiency. My parents were sympathetic, but I was told, "it's hard for some girls," and I didn't want to be seen as a wimp.

In college, I got on the pill, and things were better. But later, when I stopped taking the pill, the suppression that it provided ended, and I returned to excruciating periods.

At the time, I read a tiny snippet in an "Ask the Doctor" newspaper column. It described endometriosis and matched me exactly. I went to my OBGYN and said, "I think I have endometriosis." He laughed at me, and said "no way." I was 22. He said that endo was a disease of older woman. If I were 40, maybe. But he agreed to operate. I had my first laparoscopic exploratory surgery in 1977. The operative note reads, "the patient has massive endometriosis."

The lessons I learned were that:

* knowledge is power
* I could trust what I was experiencing in my own body despite what the doctor told me
* doctors don't know everything
* I could speak up for myself, and the world wouldn't end.

But then. Having been vindicated about my disease, I was out of knowledge. What should I do next? The surgery was only to diagnose; the endo itself was untouched. The doctor told me of a new miracle drug. I just had to take it, and I'd be fine.

Except I wasn't. On the medication, Danocrine, I had significant and permanent side effects. It was extremely expensive, and I was uninsured; though I took it religiously for an ironic nine months, it took only four days after stopping for all my symptoms to return.

There had to be a better way.

I threw myself into reading everything I could about endometriosis, including arcane medical texts in the university library basement. I joined a national support group, then was elected to its Board, then launched a local support group, then started to speak to other groups.

Around 1985, Nancy Petersen reached out to me. She is an RN who was helping to publicize the groundbreaking endometriosis work of Dr. David Redwine. He called for the treatment of endo to change radically, from medical suppression (which does nothing to treat the underlying disease) to surgical excision of all endometriosis. Nancy was (and is) a tireless advocate and mentor who sees her role as that of educator. "Each one, teach one" is her often-heard mantra.

Nancy recommended me for the extraordinary opportunity to become the founding program director for what is now an internationally-known program, the Center for Endometriosis Care (CEC) in Atlanta. To develop the program, I spent countless hours on the phone and at the computer and gave presentations all over the country, in church basements, and in enormous auditoriums. The settings were different, but the questions were always the same:

- What is wrong with me?
- Why don't my (family, friends, partner, physician) believe me?
- Why aren't there more doctors helping?

People with endometriosis were starving for information. My approach to advocacy was to lay out the facts, encourage all the questions, and then stand back to let people draw their own conclusions. I told them that we all need to become active participants in our healthcare decisions, instead of waiting, passive and afraid, for a physician to tell us the plan. I wanted to help overcome the barriers that stood between pain and resolution, and engender ownership of each individual's approach to their own healthcare issues.

The CEC, with Dr. Robert Albee and later Dr. Ken Sinervo, became wildly successful. The feedback loop between educating and empowering patients, watching them hire experts to be on their healthcare teams, and then zooming through surgery and recovery to go on to solid, fulfilling lives was enormously gratifying. It remains the best work I have ever done.

Over the past several years, I have been an Admin for the Facebook group, Nancy's Nook. As such, I've watched membership explode from a few hundred to nearly 50,000 members worldwide. During that time, the focus of the group has shifted from that of an online support group to that of an online reference library. Members are encouraged to study more than one hundred files created by the Admins to cover most aspects of endometriosis. They are then informed and empowered to work with outstanding surgeons (a curated list is maintained) and to challenge those less skilled or less aware.

It is a testament to the value of the group that many new members report their physicians/NPs/PTs sent them to join. The best doctors are not intimidated by knowledgeable patients.

It's been more than 40 years since I first heard the term "endometriosis." What has changed since then? On the positive side, some doctors are welcoming patients who know about their disease, who are forthright about their needs and who are unwilling to be fobbed off with platitudes and patronizing attitudes. Some people with endometriosis are speaking up and speaking out about their disease and their treatments. Celebrities are acknowledging that they have endo (with mixed results, to be sure), when 40 years ago that would have been career suicide.

At the same time, large pharmaceutical firms spend millions advertising medications that do not solve the problem, but are expensive and often cause significant side effects. Although the average OBGYN sees endo in their practice, few are skilled in recognizing all appearances of the disease, and fewer still are adept at its complete removal. And many of the old, outdated notions are still out there:

- just suck it up; it's only your period
- just have a baby
- just take these meds
- just have multiple surgeries, and then ...
- just have a hysterectomy.

Sigh.

Are we there yet? Hardly, but I have witnessed remarkable progress, and I am hopeful. Talking about a menstrual issue is no longer a forbidden subject, mentioning ovaries and pelvic pain is no longer conducted in whispers, if at all. I hope that 40 years from now, advocates for people with endometriosis will be an almost forgotten memory because the need for us will have vanished. xo

1

WRITING MY BODY, WRITING MY HEALTH

A Rhetorical Autoethnography

Kim Hensley Owens

When I was a sophomore in college, taking notes in a Near Eastern studies class one Tuesday afternoon, my right hand suddenly became numb and cramped. A dedicated student, I shook out my hand, glared at it, and hastily shifted to taking notes with my left hand, assuming whatever was going on with my right hand would go away. Instead, it worsened over the next few weeks. I had to quit my job at a local deli/grill because I could no longer perform the chopping, cutting, and assembling duties required. Within a few weeks, life was back to normal: I had a new job as a waitress and was able to write with my right hand again. While I can remember all of this now, after having read journal entries that jogged my memory, I had completely forgotten about this episode for years and didn't rediscover this moment from my past until I read those journals a long time after many years of (probably-related) struggle I experienced (and occasionally still do) in graduate school with shooting pains and numbness in both hands, wrists, and arms. My writing about that seemingly isolated health event in college helped me to process a scary and painful experience at the time, and later, it allowed me to piece together a timeline of causation that has helped me to better understand my body and the repetitive stress injuries it seems particularly prone to experiencing.

This chapter aims to bring readers into the lived experience of various health issues in a "feeling and embodied way" (Ellis, & Bochner, 2006, p. 437) and to elucidate the rhetorical value of health-related writing. I revisit and analyze my writing about health issues, employing what rhetorician Lunceford (2015) calls "rhetorical autoethnography." Readers of rhetorical autoethnography are invited "to 'see' the work as it happened" (p. 7). Because of the personal context provided alongside rhetorical artifacts and analysis, readers can "more fully understand the rhetorical artifact[s] under consideration" (p. 10).

In this rhetorical autoethnography, I describe and analyze snapshots of my life and writing from moments when I was consumed by heightened physical (and often accompanying emotional) pain or intensity. Following the principles laid out by Lunceford (2015), my aim is to let readers connect to me as both a writer and as an embodied being, while adding to understandings of disparate rhetorical artifacts (pp. 7–10). I rely on the scholarly traditions of autoethnographic books (e.g., Behar, 2014; Paget, & DeVault, 1993), diary analysis (e.g., Bunkers, & Huff, 1996; Gannet, 1992; Sinor, 2002), and medical and health rhetorics (e.g., Santos, 2011; Scott, 2003; Segal, 2005) to make rhetorical sense of two decades of my own health-related personal and public writing. In what follows, I focus on my writing about and advocacy for different physical issues over the last two decades of my life in a series of what might be termed analytical vignettes, or short, self-reflexive stories and analyses.

Through these analytical vignettes, I explore the functions, forms, and value of various examples of my writing about a wide range of medical issues and often-invisible-to-others challenges, including the crippling and almost career-ending wrist issues alluded to above; breast lumps, biopsies, and maternal breast cancer history; and a hip labral tear and subsequent surgery. My analysis shows that personal health-related writing allows a patient–writer to take control of her health narrative, to come to specific beliefs and understandings about her health, and to determine what actions are necessary. I argue that even private self-sponsored writing is a form of activism because it enables and distills a writer's orientation to activist thought and because it presages and provides a template for public activism.

* * *

I've been writing about my health and body for as long as I can remember, starting with diary entries from the age of ten. I've written for an audience of one about pains and kisses and joys and fears, but I haven't always written about my health and body for a more public audience. Even when I did, ostensibly, try to write for an audience, I didn't follow through on the public part at first. At 23, after undergoing surgery to have three "suspicious but probably not cancer"[1] breast lumps removed and biopsied—a procedure helpfully referred to for a young, fearful, single woman as a "partial mastectomy"—I wrote an essay of a few thousand words. After titling the piece "Triple Biopsy at Twenty-Three," I popped into a Borders bookstore to look up how to submit an article to a magazine. Following the generic submission instructions, I typed the title, my name, my address, and a word count onto a cover page, printed the essay, paper-clipped it together, and promptly placed it in a file folder, never to be sent out to anyone, ever.

Into that essay I poured every detail of the indignity of sliced-open young breasts; the enormous (to my eyes then), raised, and initially glowing-red scars; the exquisite stabs of pain I felt as I wrote on the chalkboard for the 8th grade classes I was teaching or as I zipped my breasts each morning into an infantilizing Mickey

Mouse bra—the only one I'd been able to find in stores in that pre-Amazon era when instructed to buy a "zip-up sports bra." I wrote of my near-certainty that no one would fall in love with the version of me who had such vivid scars, such visible physical flaws. While I desperately needed to write about and wanted to share my fears, pain, and worries, and while I actively imagined an audience beyond myself—a magazine-reading 20–40ish female audience, to be specific—I never actually sought one. Instead, every few months, then every year, I'd pull out the paper-clipped essay and re-immerse myself in the fears and pain associated with the experience. Later, once my fears finally proved unfounded, I'd re-read with different eyes and tried to forgive myself for melodrama.

That essay functioned similarly to a diary entry, in both the private and female-gendered forms Gannet (1992) describes as the flip sides of public and commonly male writing. However, the essay's form, with its carefully followed submission guidelines, hints at a yearning to speak to a larger audience than the audience it reached—the audience of selves (present and future) a diary typically targets. Beyond its function as a private record, the essay served the emotional purposes Pennebaker and Chung (2011) have repeatedly shown such writing can, by providing relief from the trauma. Writing the piece helped to enable an acceptance, over time, of the scare and scarring the surgery manifested. It provided a space for me to write about my experience from the inside, but also allowed me to look at my experience from the outside—allowed me first to hide from the experience in the moment, and later to re-inhabit and re-examine the experience from a different perspective, through a longer lens of time.

Most importantly, for the purposes of this autoethnographic exploration of activist health rhetorics, I drew on that piece when I first shared health information publicly. As a graduate student six or so years after the initial surgical biopsies, I had undergone additional biopsies—needle biopsies that time, with far less physical trauma involved. With my first biopsies, the emotional impact was enormous, but the financial impact nonexistent because the HMO insurance provided through my K-12 district employer had left me with a zero-dollar co-pay for surgery. My later biopsy experience in graduate school came with far less emotional drama, but with unexpected financial trauma. My graduate TA insurance coverage and the hospital's charges differed by several hundred dollars per procedure, leaving me with a bill in the thousands. My efforts to negotiate the prices with the hospital based on the "usual and customary" charges my insurance would cover were utterly unsuccessful. I learned that the term "usual and customary" has no correspondence whatsoever with the amount a provider might charge, and it made me angry.[2]

Spurred by the anger I felt at the injustice of the charging system and at the insurance that didn't cover my needs, I wrote a speech for a graduate student union rally. I knew I would be facing a crowd of mostly ambivalent fellow graduate students—some members of our then-unrecognized union, others prospective union members. I wanted to encourage my peers and colleagues to vote for a union that could negotiate to improve our insurance coverage. I began the speech by calling attention to graduate students' typical youth and presumption of good health before turning to my own story, which I started by yelling, "Do I look healthy to you?" through a bullhorn. While I now question the assumptions I asked others to make by asking that question, it was, at the time, the best way I could think of to begin to make the invisible visible. I wanted to set up the contrast between a person who might appear perfectly healthy, but nevertheless have expensive medical costs—a person who could as easily be any of them—as a reason to vote for better healthcare.

Without the diary and essay writing that preceded that speech, I would not have had the clarity of memory nor the surety of purpose to write and give the speech. The speech was my first public rendering of my own health experiences and my first action in support of collective bargaining rights. Health writing and activism were entangled, co-determining my paths as a person and as a writer.

★ ★ ★

I was in my late twenties and a couple of years into my graduate studies when, suddenly, using my fingers, hands, wrists, and forearms became excruciatingly painful. At a loss, I desperately cataloged the pain in diary entries over the next few years. I intersperse samples of these entries here to illustrate the ubiquity and range of entries and to mirror the way the pain constantly interrupted my life and thoughts.[3]

> 3 Sept. 2003: "Wrists are bad, but tendonitis is definitely keeping me from wasting time online, so that's a benefit of the pain, I guess."

Sinor (2002) probes the sparse writing of her ancestor Annie's journal to explicate its value for writing scholars. She illustrates how Annie's entries, such as those that describe wildly different kinds of events in "syntactically and physically identical" manners, illustrate how "the writer modulates how events unfurl" (p. 163). Sinor notes that studying ordinary writing allows scholars to "trac[e] how dominant discourses are internalized as well as subverted" (p. 89). Similarly, studying my journal entries—my ordinary writing—about this "wrist issue," as I often called it, allows me to trace how I internalized and/or subverted dominant discourses.

> 15 Sept. 2003: "Physical therapy (Mettler method) left me in quite a bit of pain and not a little grumpy today. The result of the PT is almost like a sunburn—a bad one—and although last week I felt better despite that surface pain, today I didn't notice much improvement, so that was frustrating."

I worked to subvert the dominant discourse that pain would impede my progress, even as I internalized the narrative that the pain might win. The pain did win, to some degree, persisting for years and interfering with not only writing and teaching, but also every aspect of daily life, from buttoning a shirt to changing channels on remote controls to holding a cup. Reading these entries forces me to remember not just the pain I felt, but to re-inhabit the spikes of hope and despair it wrought.

> 21 Sept. 2003: "I started doing the exercises in the book *How to Ease Your Carpal Tunnel Pain Without Surgery* ... it's doing very good things for me so far!"

A campus doctor—a woman from India with an accent I loved—diagnosed tendonitis and offered wrist braces, anti-inflammatories, and pain medications, but none of those helped. I dutifully wore wrist braces to work and so constantly had to answer questions about carpal tunnel syndrome—which I had been tested for and did not have, but which everyone assumed I had. Even my father would suggest that I "just have the surgery already," as if having surgery for an ailment I did not have would be logical, helpful, or even financially feasible. For six weeks, I went to physical therapy, which briefly helped. I tried acupuncture at $50 a session, which did nothing except dissipate my fear of acupuncture. I tried various forms of yoga, moist heating pads, and supplements. Even taking weeks-long breaks from doing any writing at all would provide little relief.

> 17 Dec. 2003: "Won't write too much because of wrist issues—flaring up because I've been working on final papers, argh. Still a problem/painful—I feel like I never write anymore!"

My early entries reveal attempts to find silver linings (less time wasted online!) and my early experiments with various possible solutions. I detailed the pain, the triggers, the challenges, what was working, what was not. In the first year, the entries still sounded hopeful, but by the end of that first year, frustration became the common thread—I described flare-ups; I whined; I complained about not being able to write.

> 3 March 2004: "Composing process completely mucked up by this wrist thing."

The entries settled into a series of short complaints, sometimes as an entire day's entry, contrasted with the typical multi-page monologues I would write before this issue started. The entries are short because writing by hand hurt even more than typing; they consisted of complaints because chronic pain causes chronic discouragement; by that point, a year had gone by. All manner of attempts to solve the problem had led to no discernible improvement.

> 23 June 2004: "Not-so-good hand day."

I reached the point where I felt I would have to drop out of graduate school, but returning to my fallback career of high school teaching seemed out of reach too, as the physicality of reading, writing, holding papers and holding writing implements of any kind was excruciating. Without a workable alternative life plan, I stayed in school. At this point, four-word entries became common in my diary. I recorded nothing about my life—except for pain—for weeks, months.

27 Sept. 2004: "My arms're killing me."

I managed to get through coursework; I managed to prepare for and pass my preliminary exams, but every day was an adventure in pain, pain management, and managing expectations.

10 March 2005: "My wrists are not good, which makes me not want to/ unable to work, which makes me feel guilty. When I do work ... I can't rely on freewriting because my wrists hurt ..."

Despite the pain of writing and the impediments to my usual writing processes, though, I kept writing—both the diary entries I wrote for myself and the papers I had to write as a student.

One semester I wanted to write a seminar paper on *kairos* for an Ancient Rhetorics class, but my pain was such that I couldn't think properly and felt I could not physically research what I'd planned. I had begun using voice recognition software as a way to avoid typing and to prevent more pain, and I used that experience to write a seminar paper about my challenges of writing [a seminar paper] in pain. I wrote the paper about the convergence of the physical challenges of not being able to write with the ways process writing pedagogies had contributed to my pain, about the ways that pain was making me reconsider what I was learning about ancient rhetorics, about the ways that pain was making me think about my own pedagogies. A paragraph from an early draft survives in the article that grew from it:

My experiences using three different voice recognition software programs have led me to see that moving from manual writing/typing to "oral writing" is not unproblematic, perhaps especially for those who, like me, have learned to "write" using keyboards. The injury that has led to my being unable to write/type was brought about by pedagogies, technological capabilities, and production expectations unique to my time. The software that enables this paper to be both spoken and written simultaneously is also unique to my time. I have learned to compose through writing—as a physical process including such steps as freewriting, drafting, cutting and pasting, revising, editing—and not through speaking.

(Hensley Owens, 2010)

Writing about what I was experiencing and linking that experience to what I was studying enabled me to complete a seminar paper at a time when writing seemed impossible. Thinking about my experience in terms of rhetorical and pedagogical theories also expanded my understanding.

While I now have the benefit of hindsight—as well as improved bodily awareness brought about by the Alexander Technique, the alternative therapy that eventually helped relieve most of my pain and helped me regain most function—what strikes me now about the writing I did about my wrist pain during that period is how it eventually helped me as a student and scholar. The diary entries that felt like random spurts of complaint and attempts to process pain proved critical: I read them the way one might read reference material as I constructed that seminar paper. My personal writing about my health issue ended up fueling my scholarly production. That seminar paper, written as a response to pain and as a last resort, solved the problem of necessary scholastic production in a tight timeframe for a class, but it also did far more. It strengthened my *ethos* with my professor and advisor; it provided the text for a conference presentation; it served as the first draft of what became my first accepted article; and it became the "forthcoming publication" line on my CV that helped me secure my first tenure-track job.

Writing about my health problem and exploring it in the context of the field and in terms of possibilities and limitations for myself and others allowed me to turn a medical problem into a form of self-advocacy. Beyond self-advocacy, because it explicitly argues about the potential implications and physical detriment of various pedagogical practices and the practical challenges of seemingly simple solutions, the published piece serves a more public advocacy function. I would not ask to experience the level of pain and disability I did as a graduate student again, but using writing to deal with that pain led me to research and produce scholarship that has been a boon to my career and my sense of self. Writing was a form of advocating both for pedagogical awareness and alternative solutions to health issues.

★ ★ ★

When suffering from a labral tear in my hip—a degenerative issue stemming from no clear or single source, but likely a combination of excessive use/overstretching from soccer, yoga, and my blessed genes—I wrote a long blog post comparing my mostly-hidden injury to the mostly-hidden trauma of those profiled on the television show "Hoarders." By writing that blog post, I was unknowingly doing precisely what psychological researchers Pennebaker and Chung (2011) might suggest. They note that research finds "people are most likely to benefit [from writing about trauma] if they can write a coherent story" (p. 430).

I wrote about both the invisibility of the issue, which often was just tremendous pain, and the visibility, when I needed crutches to make walking bearable but had no brace or cast or obvious-to-others reason to need them:

I look fine. I don't even usually walk noticeably strangely most of the time, though I know my gait is different, not quite right. People have no idea what's going on in my hip. And when I have to use a crutch, or two crutches, to take the pressure off sometimes, to make it possible to move from Point A to Point B, I'm embarrassed. It's strange to use a crutch, and strangely difficult to force myself to use it when I know I should but would really rather not. I see people look at me, look at the crutch, look at my feet and my legs, searching for some visual clue as to what's going on. Sometimes they ask, and I stutter out something about my hip, and they look away. Hips are embarrassing. Problems with hips seem to signal old age or infirmity in ways problems with other body parts don't. I'm 39. I shouldn't be this old yet.

(Hensley Owens, 2014)

"Hips are embarrassing," I wrote, and for the first time understood one reason why that particular bodily issue was so horrifying to me, and seemingly to others too, far beyond the physical pain. My great-grandmother died after she fell and broke her hip. Learning of her broken hip and death are two of my earliest memories. In high school, a boy I had a crush on told me his grandmother had fallen and broken her hip—I expected she would die as a result, and though I didn't tell him that, I was right. That same story could be told of countless other grandmothers. Hip issues felt *old*; they heralded death; they seemed unbearably gendered; they announced the end of vitality. And yet the kind of hip injury I had, according to my many doctors, affects mostly "active people in their late thirties and forties"—the damaged hip, to me a symbol of frailty and old age, was a symbol of contradictions: Of youth (to physicians) and middle/"old" age (to me), of activity (cause of pain) and inactivity (result of pain). The dual sides of these interpretations weren't clear to me until I wrote the post—a piece of writing that helped me in more ways than I can articulate.

Simply writing it proved to be a tremendous relief of the emotional pressure of the physical pain. Pennebaker and Chung (2011) write, "when people transform their feelings and thoughts about personally upsetting experiences into language, their physical and mental health often improve" (p. 418). That blog post fits well in the vein of expressive writing for psychological benefits. Beyond the benefits of writing for the self, though, sharing the post, which I did on Facebook, enabled me to communicate my mostly-invisible issue to dozens of people I would not have told in person, which in turn resulted in expressions of empathy, offers of concrete help (including the cadre of friends who organized dinners for my family for weeks after my eventual hip surgery), and shared stories and commiseration about physical issues friends were experiencing.

While not activism in the sense of directly attempting to affect policies or politics, a blog post like my hip post performs a kind of micro-activism. Micro-activism, like other forms of rhetorical ingenuity, lays a foundation, or cracks open a window that can lead to the empathy or understanding that precedes helpful action or public activism. Sharing the varied effects of a health issue in a personal, narrative, and emotionally raw manner is an act of micro-activism that enables an audience to inhabit, to some degree, the writer's afflicted mind and body, which strengthens the reader's ability to empathize and better understand that issue.

Empathy and understanding are critical antecedents to any form of action or activism. On an individual scale, action might include acknowledgment of the issue, expressions of empathy, and/or offers of help—small actions that are profoundly valuable for the suffering individual. On a broader scale, depending on the topic, those who read a health narrative that functions as a form of micro-activism are better-prepared and better-positioned to develop the understanding and empathy that could inspire them to engage in civic acts—from voting to letter-writing to simply telling others the story—that could help inspire preventative policies or provide support for people in similar situations.

★ ★ ★

Advocacy through personal, health-related writing can take many forms. Sometimes that advocacy is direct, as when calling a legislator or negotiating with insurance companies, and sometimes that advocacy is subtle, indirect. One such example is a snippet of personal health-related writing with an indirect-but-distinct twinge of advocating for alternative medical knowledges and practitioners in an article I wrote when I was 35. The focus of the article is rhetorics of e-health and consumer–patients, but embedded within a mostly non-narrative piece is this personal story—a story with a clear point of view:

> In a relatively healthy life, I have visited doctors far more often to learn that they cannot help me than to learn that they can. I have learned that to visit a doctor is to pay a fee for (limited) time, sometimes for information or knowledge, often for care, but rarely for "cure." By contrast, I have learned that to visit the Internet is to discover, often on the unsanctioned sites, information that can and has vastly improved my quality of life. I have learned, too, that to visit "alternative" care providers (e.g., a lay midwife, a nurse midwife, and Alexander Technique teachers) is to pay a fee for time, sometimes for information, always for care, often for "knowledge" and sometimes for "cure."
>
> (Hensley Owens, 2011, p. 228)

The author of that article was notably more skeptical about mainstream medicine than the author of this chapter is now. At 35, I had not yet been the recipient of the various fairly miraculous mainstream medical fixes I have had in the intervening years—an asthma diagnosis and medication that made breathing and moving possible and not panic-inducing after a move to a different climate revealed the illness I'd never known I had; the hip surgery that successfully repaired a labral tear that had made simply existing excruciating, the ankle ligament surgery that restored function and let me hike again after months of immobility. The author of that article had at that point only experienced repeated disappointment in mainstream medicine, and had found significant relief from alternative sources of health information and treatment, ranging from solving debilitating wrist issues in graduate school to two very healthy and happy home births.[4]

The advocacy for alternative ways of knowing that threads throughout that excerpt and the entire piece is not something I would disavow now, but I am far more open to medical ways of knowing now than I was then, and might advocate somewhat differently now. My personal experiences with medicine and health up to that point in my life colored my arguments and interpretations in ways specific to that *kairotic* moment. In the context of a rhetorical autoethnography, the above excerpt provides a snapshot; it preserves my thinking at a particular time and helps me to understand how my choices were and are circumscribed by what has come before, both long- and short-term.

One discovery from this project is that my ability to advocate for myself as a patient or medical consumer is inextricable from my ability to articulate for myself—in writing—what a physical challenge is and what it means to me. These ways of learning, being, and knowing provide a foundation for health care advocacy for the self as well as for others. The writings I've interrogated in this piece share particular commonalities—a combination of personal and private writing with an effort to reach an audience beyond myself; a focus on working through a medical crisis or diagnosis; a seeking of some kind. One describes dealing with the aftermath of medical interventions; one focuses on the challenges of not finding a medical solution, but resolves with an alternative solution; one finds hope in a medical path; one contrasts challenges of medical help with benefits of alternative health help. Each functions as advocacy to some extent, but the forms and desired outcomes of advocacy are not particularly consistent.

★ ★ ★

Breasts. Wrists. Hips. Surgeons as destroyers. Surgeons as saviors. Losing with insurance companies. Winning with insurance companies. Scars visible. Scars invisible. Problems created. Problems solved. Evolutions and explorations and complications and contradictions. My writing about my health across the last 20 years includes all of these and more. As Sinor (2002) notes, authors of ordinary texts assume varied positions and create multifaceted cultural scripts, inviting readers to "watch how cultures are made, remade, and finally ensconced in 'memory'" (p. 89). My own ordinary texts—some ordinary in the ephemeral or everyday sense Sinor explicitly invokes, and some ordinary in that they are regular aspects of an active academic's life—do this kind of work in terms of making, remaking, and remembering not only moments of embodiment and physicality, but also moments and forms of health advocacy. As forms of micro-activism, as precursors of and inspiration for further activism, they are rhetorically ingenious.

Notes

1 "probably not cancer, but ..." were the words I attributed to the doctor in my January 21, 1998 journal entry, the day I had the ultrasound that determined I would need surgical biopsies to ensure the lumps weren't cancerous.

2 For a detailed exploration of medical fees and their complicated or nonexistent relationship with the actual cost of procedures or with insurance coverage, see Brill (2013).
3 I deliberately set out even very short quotes from my diary in this section, in conscious defiance of usual citation expectations, because the interspersed entries are intended to (slightly) disrupt the reader's progress and provide a visual cue as to the constancy of the entries and constant pain.
4 For an autoethnography of my childbirth experiences, see the final chapter of Hensley Owens (2015).

References

Behar, R. (2014). *The vulnerable observer: Anthropology that breaks your heart*. Boston, MA: Beacon Press.

Brill, S. (2013). "Bitter pill: Why medical bills are killing us." *TIME.com*. Retrieved from http://content.time.com/time/subscriber/article/0,33009,2136864,00.html

Bunkers, S.L., & Huff, C.A. (Eds.). (1996). *Inscribing the daily: Critical essays on women's diaries*. Amherst, MA: University of Massachusetts Press.

Ellis, C.S., & Bochner, A.P. (2006). "Analyzing analytic autoethnography: An autopsy." *Journal of Contemporary Ethnography*, 35(4), 429–449.

Gannett, C. (1992). *Gender and the journal: Diaries and academic discourse*. Albany, NY: State University of New York Press.

Hensley, K.E. Diary excerpts, 1998–2005. Unpublished.

Hensley, K.E. (1998). Triple biopsy at twenty-three. Unpublished manuscript.

Lunceford, B. (2015). "Rhetorical Autoethnography." *Journal of Contemporary Rhetoric*, 5, 1–20.

Hensley Owens, K. (2010). "'Look Ma, no hands!': Voice-recognition software, writing, and ancient rhetoric." *Enculturation*, 7.

Hensley Owens, K. (2011). "Rhetorics of e-Health and information age medicine: A risk-benefit analysis." *JAC: A Journal of Rhetoric, Politics, and Culture*, 225–235.

Hensley Owens, K. (2014). "Invisible piles." *Kimship*. Retrieved from https://kimship. wordpress.com/2014/04/30/invisible-piles

Hensley Owens, K. (2015). *Writing childbirth: Women's rhetorical agency in labor and online*. Carbondale, IL: Southern Illinois University Press.

Paget, M.A., & DeVault, M.L. (1993). *A complex sorrow: Reflections on cancer and an abbreviated life*. Philadelphia, PA: Temple University Press.

Pennebaker, J.W., & Chung, C.K. (2011). "Expressive writing: Connections to physical and mental health." In H.S. Friedman (Ed.). *Oxford handbook of health psychology*, New York: Oxford University Press, pp. 417–437.

Santos, M. (2011). "How the Internet saved my daughter and how social media saved my family." *Kairos*, 15(2). Retrieved from http://kairos.technorhetoric.net/15.2/topoi/santos/internet_saved_my_daughter.pdf

Scott, J.B. (2003). *Risky rhetoric: AIDS and the cultural practices of HIV testing*. Carbondale, IL: Southern Illinois University Press.

Segal, J. (2005). *Health and the rhetoric of medicine*. Carbondale, IL: Southern Illinois University Press.

Sinor, J. (2002). *The extraordinary work of ordinary writing: Annie Ray's diary*. Iowa City, IA: University of Iowa Press.

2

TEMPORAL DISRUPTIONS

Illness Narratives Before and After Web 2.0

Ann Wallace

I had just turned 22 in March 1992, two months shy of college graduation, when a nurse practitioner felt a large mass in my abdominal cavity. Within weeks, I underwent a battery of diagnostic tests, had surgery to remove a massive teratoma, was diagnosed with ovarian cancer, and began chemotherapy. My hair fell out from under my mortarboard as I walked across the stage that May to receive my diploma. I graduated into a world very different from the one my classmates were entering. Two days later, I shaved my head and buckled down for a summer marked by needles strewn across my coffee table, bags of chemotherapy in my refrigerator, and thrice weekly visits from home healthcare nurses.

The displacement into the realm of illness is as total as it is uncertain, layered with impossible questions about treatment, prognosis, and recovery. Life with cancer in 1992, at a time when people still lowered their voices to utter the dreaded two syllables, when internet health sites and support groups did not yet exist, when showing a bare head invited unwelcomed stares, sympathy, and even ridicule, was easiest when I stayed focused each day on making it through to the next, no more and no less. An art student in college, I had visions of creating a popup public installation of a cancer house and of collaborating with a friend on a comic strip entitled *Chemo Chic*; yet, even as I imagined these modest projects, I knew that they would never be realized.

When feminist literary scholar Susan Gubar was diagnosed with ovarian cancer in 2008, she felt profoundly calm. Despite her dire prognosis, she recalls "a pervasive sense of release," as the diagnosis came after weeks spent in medical limbo, during which, as she put it, "my window to the world began to be fogged or curtained so I could only intermittently peer through its gauzy veil as I emigrated from the world of the healthy to the domain of the ill" (Gubar, 2012, p. 5). Diagnosis provided a simultaneously frightening and illuminating metaphorical line of clarity separating Gubar's past from her present with finality. Segal (2005) similarly situates diagnosis as a discursive construction that we rely on to make sense of time and space; "we crave diagnoses" (p. 116). Diagnosis provides clarity—even when it comes with a dire prognosis.

I know Gubar's feeling well as I have twice been handed a diagnosis that was unexpected in both its severity and its specificity: When I learned that I had ovarian cancer, and many years later in 2009, when I was diagnosed with MS. However, the experience of facing a deadly form of cancer as a young woman in the 1990s was markedly different from becoming an MS patient as I neared the age of 40 in the post-millennial age. I have come to realize that these distinctions, though impacted by age and experience, arise mainly from the recent, exciting shift in the rhetoric of illness and of illness narratives more specifically. Rather than medical advances, changes in cultural-discursive responses to illness have made facing MS now an entirely more communal experience for me than living through cancer in 1992 was. Today, expanding roles available to me as audience and as patient make living through a difficult diagnosis less isolating, and my sense of community comes from the ability to share my experiences online.

In this essay, I critically examine these two periods of my life side by side and put them into sociohistorical context by drawing upon the work of poet Marilyn Hacker and queer literary theorist Eve Kosofsky Sedgwick—both diagnosed with breast cancer in the early 1990s—to help situate my cancer experience within its rhetorical moment which, I argue, was heavily shaped by the AIDS pandemic and the rise of breast cancer advocacy. I, then, move forward in time to consider how Gubar's and my own response to post-millennial diagnoses have rhetorical, if not genre-based, similarities that bespeak very different cultural understandings of illness, which I attribute to important discursive shifts in online authoring practices in Web 2.0. I ultimately argue that women's online health narratives, which have analogs in earlier print publications of women's health and witnessing experiences, constitute rhetorical ingenuity since these everyday texts adeptly imagine audiences at various temporal stages—diagnosed, in treatment, recovering, dying, or in mysterious symptoms limbo—with raw immediacy.

Indeed, while the 1980s–1990s were charged with the politics of silence—death, of debunking stigmatizing metaphors of illness, and of bringing humanity and visibility to those facing so-called shameful diseases—the past two decades or so have been marked by a preponderance of cancer stories, written with raw immediacy for audiences of responsive readers armed with a wealth of online health information. Very little causes these experienced readers to flinch, yet Gubar's story, like other women's health narratives, has the capacity to unsettle as she traces the emotional upheaval of arriving at a diagnosis and commits to writing the story many little-known online writers have written—a story that she composes while she believes she is dying and that she presents, largely unfiltered, for her audience while in medical and existential limbo.

Like others narrating their illness stories, Gubar (2012) makes it clear that her cancer diagnosis signals the move from what Sontag had identified decades earlier as "the kingdom of the well" to "the kingdom of the sick" (p. 3). It is striking that Sontag's argument still resonates in the post-millennial era, years after Web 2.0 authoring seems to have lifted the silencing veil on illness narratives. Segal (2005) argues that fetishizing diagnosis as *the* essential answer in a quest for health is common. A diagnosis disrupts one's sense of identity at the most elemental level as the diagnosis becomes the final word. Gubar (2016) confirms the sense of finality, explaining that "Hearing a diagnosis is, in other words, shock, and injury … and a threshold: One stage of life has closed; another is opening. We wander between two worlds, one extinct and the other frightfully unpredictable" (p. 17). Indeed, many survivors divide their lives into Before Cancer and After Cancer, as diagnosis still metaphorically demarcates the end of one life and beginning of another.

Something held me back from my artistic impulses in the early 1990s, something I could not name until I picked up a copy of Sontag's (1990) *Illness as Metaphor* the following year. I had not been able to speak past my fear of others' discomfort in the face of the mortality of a young woman speaking from one kingdom, of the ill, to the other, where people do not have IVs in their arms or wear scarves and hats to cover their bald heads. I refused to hide the signs of my cancer, but I could not take on the added task of telling my story.

Thankfully, however, bold writers did tell their stories, and as web authoring opened up to new voices, possibilities for composing unspeakable narratives expanded dramatically. When I found myself with MS, then, there were far more readily available avenues through which I could share my new realities in temporally complicated ways. These new platforms for illness stories, of course, retain traces of previous eras even as they constitute new writing terrain.

Writing Elegies in an Age of Death

At the height of the seemingly his-and-her pandemics of AIDS and breast cancer in the 1980s, telling the story of disease was a radical act. As men and women died at alarming rates, they too often did so in silence and alone, unable to break past the imposed stigma. Yet by the start of the 1990s, many allied writers deliberately took on the work of bearing witness from positions of health, and these writers carved out space for other writers to compose narratives from positions of illness later on. Hacker (1994) and Sedgwick (1993) commemorate their friends' and loved ones' lives and focus on the individual stories of illness and untimely death while simultaneously commenting on the impact of an epidemic. The deaths that surround them mark a generation, and, as witnesses, they struggle to find ways to make meaning of their compounding losses. Dawes (1995) gestures to their struggles when he explains that counting and naming are two different acts; when we are confronted with the enormity, the individual is lost (p. 30). The most impactful memorials, however, are able to recognize both—such as the Names Project AIDs

Memorial Quilt, which grew to such immense proportions that it was displayed in its entirety on the Washington Mall. In the Quilt, the specific and the collective exist together, as bodies are transformed into panels, which Howe (1997) posits are stitched together into the "novelistic enterprise" of piecework mourning and commemoration (p. 112).

It is in this spirit that Hacker and Sedgwick wrestle with their roles as survivors of the AIDs crisis. They build upon the traditional elegiac form, looking beyond the individual life to interweave the dying with the well, victims with survivors, and thus challenging linear and singular temporalities. Literal witnessing expands with metaphorical vision as they record the trauma of the epoch, inviting readers to see the suffering and loss. Each stanza, each line, functions much like a panel within the Quilt—upsetting on its own, but devastating when juxtaposed.

In "Against Elegies," Hacker (1994) states bluntly, "James has cancer. Catherine has cancer. / Melvin has AIDS. / Whom will I call, and get no answer?" (p. 11). She opens with the names of those she knows, but leaves room for the nameless, "The earth-black woman in the bed beside / Lidia on the AIDS floor—deaf, and blind: / I want to know if, no, how she died." She is overwhelmed, and the stanza ends with the difficult truth, "I left her name behind" (p. 13). Similarly, Sedgwick (1993) recalls a panel from the Quilt that reads, "He hated the quilt," a nameless record of a man who resisted being memorialized, yet his panel of fabric now lies among thousands of other casket-sized panels (p. 265). These lines reveal the uneasy ways in which Hacker and Sedgwick learn to incorporate, as best they can, the trauma that they are surviving.

Sedgwick and Hacker identify themselves as survivors in the historical sense, defined by Bahar (2003) as like that of the Holocaust, as large-scale loss unfolds before them and they search for points of identification. Fuss (1995) argues that "identification works as a kind of elegy, remembering and commemorating the lost object by ritualistically incorporating its serial replacements" (p. 38).

Hacker and Sedgwick express similar commitments to bearing witness. In both women's writings, health and illness are discrete categories, and identification seems possible only when surviving allies such as Hacker and Sedgwick serve as metaphorical tour guides showing us who lived where. Yet, how firm is the line between health and illness? Zeiger (1997) claims that elegies in a time of AIDS respond to the blurring relationship between the living and the dead, the breaking down of the categories of the witness, or those at risk, and the elegized. He further argues that poetry written in memory of gay men—much like panels of the Quilt—has a dual elegiac function of simultaneously mourning the deceased and those at risk. Such blurring occurs within the work of Hacker and Sedgwick, but neither of these women thought herself to be at risk. And yet, they both are, of course, as are all of us.

The metaphor of survivor in the illness discourses of the 1990s became unsettled, in part, via medical metaphors. Segal (2005) argues that this language of survival with regards to illness has only become possible in recent years, with a shift toward patient agency within medicine. A confluence of shifts in cultural understandings—of trauma, of queer identity, of loss, of illness, of patients' agency—needed to occur in order for Marilyn Hacker's and Eve Sedgwick's expanded use of "survivor" to resonate successfully and fully, and the dynamic nature of Web 2.0 authoring made these shifts available to everyday writers.

Writing Through Illness

In 1992, I felt no compulsion to write the story of my cancer. Illness memoir was not yet a popular form, I had no ready audience, and I had not yet situated my experience within the larger moment. Instead, I went to graduate school and searched out others' sanctioned, published stories, like those cited above. I needed to understand the terrain of cancer literature, to unpack the metaphors and embodied images, to examine the appeals to readers and points of identification that inform stories of cancer. Fascinated by the ways in which writers compose themselves into a subject position, I read and wrote, while marking the remaining silences within the growing body of illness literature. One of the persistent silences I noted was my own story, that of ovarian cancer.

When Gubar was diagnosed in 2008, she too recognized the dearth of ovarian cancer narratives: "There are very few published accounts for [women with ovarian cancer] to consult since for decades, indeed for centuries, women have generally maintained silence about the silent killer" (2012, p. 2). In fact, Gubar notes at the start of her memoir (2012) that it is such a ruthless disease that 70% of women are diagnosed after the disease has spread, when it is nearly always fatal (p. 1). She posits that in their final days, women are not likely to write about the "disintegration of the body" (p. 2). Yet in the window of time Gubar believed she had, she wrote the book that she wished had been available for her, a book that unflinchingly describes the process of dying. As she cautions in the Preface to her book, "[My story] is not comforting" (p. xiii). Even so, she hopes it will "do some good work in the world" and lead to improved treatment of a disease whose survival rates have hardly changed in the past 25 years (p. xiii).

Gubar (2012) does not *want* to write *Memoir of a Debulked Woman*, but as she learns that her torturous ordeal is not unusual, her conviction to write deepens. Steeped in depression, she records that the cancer treatments "debilitate the person dealing with it until she barely recognizes her mind, spirit, or body as her own. Enduring ovarian cancer mires patients in treatments more patently hideous than the symptoms originally produced by the disease" (p. 3). This is a theme she picks up again in a chapter on chemotherapy, in which she details the compounding cognitive dissonance of treatment, employing the metaphor of torture. But chemotherapy is only one element of her pain; the invasive abdominal surgery and ongoing difficulties with her colon and bowels are so dehumanizing that Gubar describes herself in the third person as "the debulked woman" in an extended description (pp. 70–71). She is writing so close to the edge of horror that she employs a dissociative technique to distance herself as a writer. Still, she continues recording even though, "The thought of people I know and people I don't know acquiring information about the most private aspects of my life twists me in knots" (p. xvii). The imperative to create a record for others—and to do so before her predicted death—supersedes her cognitive or emotional comfort.

Gubar uses the tools honed through a career of textual analysis. When she turns herself into her subject, she lives—and writes—through a self-reflective lens. She steps back to analyze each moment not only after, but even beforehand, explaining, "If I know that I am going to record an event, like an upcoming and difficult conversation, I become more mindful about analyzing its subtleties while I engage in it. The very prospect focuses my attention" (p. 33). She is highly aware that her life is the story she is writing, and her writer's mindset guides her experience as patient. Yet it is illuminating when she comments that "Writing about cancer is not quite the same as having cancer" even as she is writing in time with her experience, using a witnessing lens to shape herself as patient, the life and the story are not identical (p. 31). But she collapses them into a nearly seamless overlap for her audience. She has one small window in which to write about cancer, as it is expected there will be no after cancer for her.

Writing against time, Gubar engages in life writing that is disorganized, raw, and immediate, that delivers unsettling information to readers without the comfort of resolution, and that, thus, disrupts everyday temporalities and the fiction of a narrative illness arc that ends in wellness. Frank (2013) argues that most illness narratives take one of three forms: Restitution, chaos, or quest (p. xiv). It is easy to identify Gubar's written account as chaotic, in which "life is reduced to a series of present-tense assaults" (Frank, 2013, p. xv). Indeed, when Gubar survives despite her doctor's dire prognosis, it escalates rather than relieves the chaos of the story, as the one seemingly sure thing, her impending death, does not happen. Frank (2013) notes that "Many people with chronic illnesses, especially MS, have written about this diagnostic uncertainty," yearning for a firm diagnosis and trajectory for their health (p. xv). I recognize the voice with which Gubar writes in the face of such uncertainty. It is much like my own in writing about MS.

Decades ago, the trajectory of my ovarian cancer was very clear: I was diagnosed in a timely manner, underwent an unimaginably grueling, but successful course of treatment, and then embarked on my adult life as a cancer survivor with a sobering sense of mortality indelibly shaped by my experience. There was no step of writing my illness; I reflected on how cancer had shaped me and shared my insights directly with my circle of friends and indirectly through my scholarly work. MS, however, has been an entirely different sort of disease; it has been, ironically, much closer to Gubar's ovarian cancer in its lack of certainty and the unending array of actual and potential debilitating symptoms, exams, and treatments. Like Gubar, I find that writing itself, as an act that requires reflection even as an event is happening, helps me to make sense of the chaos as it happens without relying upon a linear narrative that builds to a point of resolution. Of course, there is no restitution with my MS or with Gubar's cancer—and even if there might eventually be, there is none at the moment of writing.

One of the hallmarks of the 21st century and Web 2.0 is that information is shared online immediately, unceasingly, and globally. In regard to healthcare, patients have gained knowledge and agency because of these new discursive realities. Indeed, the fields of narrative medicine and RHM have arisen in line with the assertion that patients' stories have value, and patients have gained agency and audiences from peers and medical professionals alike. These stories have urgency and immediate audiences. Gubar composed her book because, as a woman ravenous for patient accounts of the illness she was facing, she could not find any. She worked in a mode familiar to her as a literary scholar even as she created a raw and open-ended memoir with no clear resolution. Today's readers, in their demand for current, of-the-moment writing, are willing to embrace a narrative that is incomplete, raw, and that takes us close to the edge.

Yet after the *Memoir of a Debulked Woman* was complete, responding to readers' demands for ever more immediate information presented in smaller, accessible doses, Gubar began writing the "Living with Cancer" blog for *The New York Times* in 2014, a composing experience she discusses at length in *Reading and Writing Cancer* (Gubar, 2016). In her blog, readers see the extent to which the rhetorical dynamic has shifted away from the authoritative expert—whether the doctor or even the memoirist—and onto the reader. Segal (2009) delves into internet health as a "bidirectional process," in which readers shape the information available (via their comments and even passively through online search terms) as much as medical information shapes them (p. 359). This is not necessarily, in her opinion, a good thing, leading to the new phenomenon of "cyberchondria," a term coined by Ryen White and Eric Horvitz in 2008, in which people arrive at extreme self-diagnoses supported by information found online (as cited in Segal, 2009, p. 361). Segal (2009) further theorizes that internet health users fall into two categories: Those seeking information on chronic conditions and those looking to self-diagnose (p. 361). Perhaps her readers' potential proclivity toward cyberchondria explains Gubar's (2016) admission that "On the internet, I failed to solve the problem of writing truthfully about my body" (p. 172). Despite the reality that "sometimes exactly what we cannot express to family and friends needs to be put down in her words" (p. 169), she does not post every blog entry she writes, withholding the most lurid ones. She posits this as modesty ("Did I really want my colleagues all around the country to know about my daily problems with poop?" [p. 165]), but she has already written a book—which presumably many of her colleagues have read—that shares far more intimate details than found in an 850-word blog. It seems more likely that Gubar feels a responsibility toward her readers; uncomfortably vivid posts have shock value that detract from her mission, fueling readers' fears rather than allaying them. Thus, Gubar brings an order and tidiness to her online writing that she willingly and truthfully jettisons in her book.

It is in this and other distinctions between the two genres—online blog post versus full-length memoir—that we can best appreciate how skillfully and deliberately Gubar handles the rhetoric of illness in the 21st century. In her memoir, she abandons an easy narrative in favor of a truthful, immediate account of a silent disease; on her blog, acutely aware of online readers' susceptibility to fear and panic, she shapes her posts to calm nerves. In both, however, she writes for the patient, current or not yet diagnosed, who yearns to better understand life with terminal cancer and find a sense of community in the process. In both, she challenges linear narrative assumptions in favor of tending to temporal uncertainty. In both, she, thus, exhibits rhetorical ingenuity.

Her project would not have been possible just 20 years earlier, when writers like Sedgwick and Hacker needed to show that the value of illness narratives outweighs readers' desire to metaphorically look away. But the proliferation of memoirs in the late 1990s created a public eager to identify with the trauma of illness and eager for an ever-closer bedside seat. Nonetheless, one is never fully prepared for the experience of being tucked into the metaphorical hospital bed oneself; I certainly was not, even after having been there before. But in the age of the internet, I was able to imagine an audience, like Gubar does, and write my way through the chaos. And as I do so, drafting poems in the emergency room or in the car after a doctor's appointment, or crafting prose pieces at home, I think of Gubar composing her illness as she lives it, unsure if she will live past it. While MS will not kill me, it is incurable, and we live in a moment that allows me to write, with confidence, about the messiness of that uncertainty. The immediacy with which information is shared in this new century has, to be sure, complicated healthcare; but it has simultaneously opened up the exciting possibility of telling a story of illness that resists a graceful arc, tidy ending, and temporal stability. And with that shift, perhaps we are able to understand illness beyond the trajectory of diagnosis to cure, and see that most of the experience of being sick exists far outside of that framework.

References

Bahar, S. (2003). "'If I'm one of the victims, who survives?': Marilyn Hacker's breast cancer texts." *Signs*, 28(4), 1025–1052.

Dawes, J. (1995). "Narrating disease: AIDS, consent, and the ethics of representation." *Social Text*, 43, 27–44.

Frank, A.W. (2013). *The wounded storyteller: Body, illness, and ethics*. Chicago, IL: University of Chicago Press.

Fuss, D. (1995). *Identification papers*. New York: Routledge.

Gubar, S. (2012). *Memoir of a debulked woman: enduring ovarian cancer*. New York: W.W. Norton & Company.

Gubar, S. (2016). *Reading and writing cancer: how words heal*. New York: W.W. Norton & Company.

Hacker, M. (1994). *Winter Numbers*. New York: W.W. Norton & Company.

Howe, L. (1997). "The AIDS quilt and its traditions." *College Literature*, 24(2), 109–124.

Sedgwick, E.K. (1993). *Tendencies*. Durham, NC: Duke University Press.

Segal, J.Z. (2005). *Health and the rhetoric of medicine*. Carbondale, IL: Southern Illinois University Press.

Segal, J.Z. (2009). "Internet health and the 21st-century patient: A rhetorical view." *Written Communication*, 26(4), 351–369.

Sontag, S. (1990). *Illness as metaphor and AIDS and its metaphors*. New York: Anchor.

Zeiger, M.F. (1997). *Beyond consolation: death, sexuality, and the changing shapes of elegy*. Ithaca, NY: Cornell University Press.

3

ANALYZING PCOS DISCOURSES

Strategies for Unpacking Chronic Illness and Taking Action

Marissa McKinley

Online health communities, or peer-to-peer Internet communities dedicated to health literacy and promotion (Willis, & Royne, 2017), provide people with an alternative space for personal health management. Within these communities, users gain access to specialized health information, emotional support, and psychosocial benefits from those who share in similar diagnoses (Dobransky, & Hargittai, 2012; Househ, Borycki, & Kushniruk, 2014; Yoo et al., 2014). Fox (2011) speaks to the popularity of online health communities, noting that one in four individuals actively participates in the communities, and of those who participate, individuals are seeking medical advice and others with whom to connect. The building of community is, partly, what makes online health communities appealing to those suffering from illness, such as women with PCOS.

PCOS is a chronic, hormonal-metabolic, genetic disorder affecting 5–10% of women in the US (US DHHS, 2016). Women with PCOS risk becoming insulin resistant due to increased production of insulin by the pancreas. With a persistent dependence on the pancreas to transport blood sugar (glucose) throughout the body, muscle and fat tissue develop increasing unresponsiveness, resulting in insulin resistance.

Due to the increase in insulin, women with PCOS also produce increased levels of androgens, typically labeled as male sex hormones. Androgens lead to the expression of physiological characteristics such as acne, obesity, hair loss, skin tags, deepening of voice, darkening of skin on the breasts and in skin folds, and excess facial and body hair (hirsutism) (US DHHS, 2016). Additionally, women with PCOS experience irregular and absent menstrual cycles, shrinking of the ovaries, and infertility (US DHHS, 2016).

At present, a cure for PCOS does not exist; however, PCOS specialists, such as endocrinologists, dermatologists, and gynecologists recommend that women with

PCOS take a proactive, multifaceted approach when managing and treating their symptoms. This includes lifestyle changes such as weight loss and exercise, birth control pills to improve regularity in ovulation and menstruation, anti-androgen drugs to manage cystic acne and hirsutism, and diabetic drugs to regulate insulin levels within the PCOS body (Barry, Kuczmierczyk, & Hardiman, 2011). Yet, even those who follow these recommendations can still feel overwhelmed by their condition and limited in their options for disease management and treatment; as a result, some will turn to online health communities, such as myPCOSteam, to seek emotional support and insights from women who share in their diagnosis.

In this chapter, I study the language practices of women diagnosed with PCOS as they participate in the free, online health forum myPCOSteam.[1] The forum provides users with a variety of sources to help them locate PCOS health specialists, as well as a space for networking and social support. Similar to the previvor blogs that Siegel Finer (2016) describes, the myPCOSteam forum helps respond to the rhetorical needs of the PCOS community. Siegel Finer defines rhetorical needs as "fillable (1) only in writing, (2) for a specific audience, and (3) for the purpose of engaging that audience rhetorically (to act)" (p. 177). As I will capture in this chapter, myPCOSteam users rely on the forum to unpack their own health experiences and to seek out medical advice from those who share their diagnosis. In so doing, myPCOSteam users fulfill their own rhetorical needs.

My analysis is influenced by muted group theory (MGT), described below, which allows me to highlight the myPCOSteam writers' engagement in practices of rhetorical ingenuity. Defined by the editors of this collection as "the practices of creating one's own rhetorical means for highly specific, often technical, and extremely personal health-related rhetorical situations" (p. 2), rhetorical ingenuity acknowledges the agency of individuals and how they construct and enact communicative strategies that allow them to operate around health systems and practices that seek to marginalize them, exemplified by the dismissive attitudes of doctors that some participants report. The writers that I discuss in this chapter come to myPCOSteam for personal reasons; often, these women share their PCOS experiences and seek advice for treating their PCOS symptoms. In a time where, each year, it becomes more and more costly to treat and manage a chronic illness like PCOS, women with limited incomes must look for alternatives outside of official healthcare systems for support and disease management. Online health communities, like myPCOSteam, fulfill this need, and it is within these spaces where users employ their rhetorical ingenuity to improve their own and others' lives.

Literature Review

Scholarship within the fields of technical communication and medical rhetoric highlights the affordances of online health communities for those suffering from an array of illnesses. Willis and Royne (2017) investigate online health communities for arthritis patients, who use them to gain knowledge related to drug management, symptom management information, and social support. Holladay (2017) investigates the practices of those participating in a mental health discussion forum, finding that writers within the digital space interpret and manipulate psychiatric information to benefit their community. These studies evidence that participants within digital health communities use the spaces to respond to their own health needs.

Research on digital health communities also indicates that the communities provide unique opportunities for women to gain emotional support and validation when it comes to their embodied health experiences. In her examination of the online health community *Breast Cancer World*, Beemer (2016) finds that women use the digital space to "gather knowledge that is born from lived experience" and to exchange discourse, which can lead to patient "empowerment and liberation" (p. 95). De Hertogh's (2015) study of the online birthing community, *Birth Without Fear*, finds that the community provides an alternative space to influence women's embodied knowledge. De Hertogh concludes that *Birth Without Fear* assists women with rewriting rhetorics tied to perceptions of their bodies and their health. These studies suggest that digital health communities can be spaces where women can work together to create a discourse of self-empowerment—a place where, through knowledge-sharing, women can support one another.

On the other hand, Pitts (2004) highlights how the Internet can be a contentious space for users. Pitts analyzes the writing produced by women with breast cancer and explores the affordances of breast cancer web pages for users. Pitts contends that while women's web pages may offer possibilities for women's knowledge construction in relation to "what are often highly political aspects of the body, gender, and illness," she reasons that the Internet is not always an "inherently empowering technology" (p. 34). She finds that the technology, in fact, may be a tool that upholds and supports the "norms of femininity, consumerism, individualism and other powerful social messages" (p. 34). Even so, the preponderance of research suggests that online health communities and especially forums like myPCOSteam offer more advantages than disadvantages for its users. The present study verifies this claim.

Methods and Methodology

This chapter examines correspondences produced by women with PCOS participating in a myPCOSteam forum, guided by two main research questions:

1. What rhetorical strategies do women with PCOS employ when participating in an online PCOS health community?
2. What can rhetoricians learn about the rhetorical strategies employed by women participating in an online PCOS health community?

Methods

To address these questions, I relied on two feminist research methodologies to underlie the collection and coding of 25 randomly selected posts on myPCOSteam in 2017.[2] To code the posts, I relied primarily on Saldaña's (2009) work on qualitative coding, selecting descriptive coding to first summarize the data. To engage in descriptive coding, Tesch (1990) recommends writing down a word or short phrase that identifies the topic—what is being "talked or written about" (p. 119)—within the content. In two rounds, I noted, organized, and summarized the general topics. The words or phrases (i.e., codes) generated after my second examination were then further combined and refined before recording them in a codebook.

Before manual coding commenced for all posts, intercoder agreement of the coding scheme was tested by a second coder versed in qualitative coding, who code three myPCOSteam posts. Intercoder agreement was then calculated for the posts. The following formula was utilized to calculate intercoder agreement: Number of agreements ÷ total number of ratings × 100 = intercoder agreement. We underwent two rounds of norming to further refine the codes we felt were problematic; on the second time, we obtained 88% intercoder agreement, which was above our target percentage of 80%. I then recorded all revised codes in a codebook before manually coding the remaining posts.

Twenty-four codes were organized under four themes. Choice phrases from the participants were then incorporated into the titles of the themes to signify the importance of the women's voices. Thus, the following themes emerged:

1. "I was diagnosed almost three years ago": Unpacking facets of health.
2. "Has anyone else …?": Taking self-action.
3. "I feel like I can't take it anymore": Emotional weight.
4. "I have facial I guess features that resemble a guy": Gesturing toward identity.

With codes organized into themes, I reviewed the data once more to note the rhetorical strategies used by participants within myPCOSteam to fulfill their own rhetorical needs when participating in the forum. In this article, I will focus my analysis on the two most predominantly coded themes.

Methodology

Two methodologies grounded my analysis. First, the methodology derived from Denzin's (1996) and Christians' (2005) Feminist Communitarian Model (FCM) suggests that research projects should serve the community being studied, rather than "the community of knowledge producers and policy makers" (Denzin, 1996, p. 275). As such, the researcher adopting the model actively works to communicate with the community being studied throughout the research process, sharing anything from the purpose(s) of the research project to the data collected and analyzed with the community. This approach "breaks down the walls between subjects and researchers" (Christians, 2005, p. 157), and, as noted by Denzin, "ought to be excluded from IRB oversight" (Denzin, 1996, p. 249). Christians asserts that while IRBs seek to protect individuals participating in research by "ensuring that informed consent is always obtained in human subject research," in reality, IRBs "protect institutions and not individuals" (2005, p. 148). From this perspective, signing an IRB does not guarantee that a subject is protected, but rather, the institution is protected. In this way, power remains with the institution in an idealized, non-mutual system, and not with the subject. If the purpose of the FCM is to be communal, mutual, and reciprocal between researcher and subject, then having subjects sign an IRB deconstructs the model, and it imposes a relationship of domination between the researcher, subject, and institution. The IRB, then, acts as a form of control and assumes that the researcher remains disinterested in "giving the group power" (Denzin, 1996, p. 243). These are not the goals, nor the values, of the FCM, which aims to promote mutuality, critical consciousness, and social transformation—aims that guided the larger research project from which this chapter originates.

To enact the FCM, ownership of the data that resulted from this larger research project was shared with myPCOSteam administrators. The data may allow the administrators to learn more about their participants, which could render understandings about how various social, environmental, and health factors potentially impact the physical health of myPCOSteam users. Equipped with this information, it is my hope that myPCOSteam administrators will introduce initiatives to help improve the health of women with PCOS.

The second arm of my methodology is Muted Group Theory (MGT), which focuses on the communication practices of dominant groups (e.g., men) and how these groups "suppress, mute, [or] devalue" (Kramarae, 2009, p. 667) the voices of subordinate groups (e.g., women and other minorities). The theory has often been used in studies focused on gender. For example, in reviewing the work of cultural ethnographers, Ardener (1975) found that the male perspective was often privileged, and research findings were frequently generalized to the male population and ignored the women. Based on this finding, Ardener reasoned that because men have historically produced and controlled language, those trained in ethnography have simply reproduced the language privileged and bounded by society—the language of men. This theory suggests that by having their words and ideas discursively reproduced, men maintain their dominance over subordinate groups, silencing their speech and thus their experiences. When the voices of men overshadow those of women, the experiences of men become seemingly ever more important, providing the marginalization of women and their decreased authority to articulate their own experiences. This study champions MGT to highlight the rhetorical ingenuity of the women who often must go outside of medical authorities to be heard and also to gain helpful information about PCOS. Considering the myPCOSteam writers through the lens of MGT for this study works to further acknowledge the importance of their strategies around health topics specific *to women by women*.

"I was diagnosed almost three years ago": Unpacking facets of health

Overwhelmingly, many of the myPCOSteam posts engage with the theme of "unpacking." In these posts, users often note when they were diagnosed, and they detail their current symptoms and treatment experiences with physicians. One user, Loren_Lasher02,[3] unpacks facets of her health by discussing her PCOS journey. She explains that she was diagnosed three years ago by a "former PCP (internal medicine NP) and a[n] OBGYN." Loren_Lasher02 further details her experiences with obesity and how, after moving to a new town and meeting with a new OBGYN, her doctor explained that if she "just lost weight," she "wouldn't have PCOS." After later meeting with another OBGYN, Loren_Lasher02 was told the same—lose weight, and your PCOS symptoms will basically vanish. Loren_Lasher02 admits that she has tried to lose weight after her healthcare visits, but she has done so "without success."

Loren_Lasher02's struggles with weight gain are not unique, for, as evidenced within the forum, other users admit to their own struggles with obesity. In her myPCOSteam post, MsVanessa14 explains how she, too, was "basically told [that she was] fat and need[ed] to lose weight" after an appointment with her healthcare provider. Like Loren_Lasher02, MsVanessa14 was not prescribed any medication to help her lose weight. Instead, and, unlike Loren_Lasher02, she was referred to a health specialist.

While obesity was one PCOS symptom that myPCOSteam users often unpacked in the forum, another PCOS symptom that was frequently discussed was infertility. For example, PrincesssLiza explains that she is on "a ton of other meds" and that her doctor wants to "add another one," even though the medications that she is taking are not helping her conceive. Her frustration is evident when she writes, "So now I need a remedy to lower the prolactin levels so I can get pregnant without a new medication." Other users also detail symptoms associated with PCOS that make conceiving difficult. EmmaLazarus discusses how she has seen "several" OBGYNs in her attempts to conceive. However, she has never been able to become pregnant due to a lack of menstrual cycles since October 2014 and thanks to a "very large fibroid." EmmaLazarus reports that several doctors have told her that she needs a hysterectomy, but she refuses to give up on becoming pregnant. EmmaLazarus hopes that seeing a reproductive endocrinologist will, one day, help her to conceive.

The words of Loren_Lasher02, MsVanessa14, PrincesssLiza, and EmmaLazarus tell a similar story: Having PCOS comes with serious health challenges. It appears that, despite seeing a variety of physicians to help them manage PCOS symptoms and to help them achieve their health goals (i.e., losing weight, conceiving), physicians are rather demeaning and unhelpful. As reported by the women, physicians tell them to simply lose weight or to have a hysterectomy without helping the women locate other treatment options. No one mentions prescriptions for Metformin—a medication that can help women with PCOS lose weight by helping the body to metabolize insulin more effectively. And there are no mentions of referrals to reproductive specialists. Instead, the women are left without further medical assistance from health experts. Left with more questions than answers about their current health status, the women turn to myPCOSteam, unpacking facets of their health to women who share in their diagnosis.

"Has anyone else …?": Taking self-action

The theme with the second largest number of codes is "Taking self-action," which consists largely of two actions: Asking questions and performing what I term self-research. In lieu of more formalized and institutional educational contexts, such as a clinical space, many of the women are either asking fellow myPCOSteam users for advice on a topic related to PCOS, or are asking for others' experiences with taking a medication. For instance, in her post, myPCOSteam user, LoraEllen, queries about others' experiences with taking Aviane birth control pills. LoraEllen begins her post by unpacking her diagnosis and states that her gynecologist has prescribed her Aviane to alleviate PCOS symptoms. She then asks, "Does anyone have any positive experience taking this to alleviate symptoms?" LoraEllen concludes her post by explaining that she will soon visit an endocrinologist to do further blood tests on her cortisol levels.

Another user, Allisa, inquires about the diabetic drug, Victoza. She wonders if anyone participating in the forum has had success with the medication. Allisa is searching for advice because her doctor is recommending the drug and because "Metformin doesn't control [her] sugars."

The women within myPCOSteam ask a variety of other questions. Robyn asks if anyone within the forum is also on the waiting list for *in vitro* fertilization. RittaL wonders if anyone else on the forum struggles with their legs itching after shaving, and she then asks for suggestions for how to stop the problem. Finally, IvetteEminda explains that two months ago, she was diagnosed with PCOS via sonogram; she admits, "I am unsure which one I have." She then inquires, "Is the OBGYN diagnose that? If so how?" Instead of consulting physicians with their questions for reasons noted above, these women are searching for answers on the myPCOSteam forum with the goal of eliciting advice from other women with PCOS. In this way, LoraEllen, Allisa, Robyn, RittaL, and IvetteEminda engage in a unique form of self-research and attempt to retrieve answers that assist them with making their own health decisions.

Another form of action that women are taking within myPCOSteam is the time to engage in self-research, not only using the Internet to look up information related to PCOS, but spreading the information to help others. This is distinct from coming to myPCOSteam simply to gain information for oneself. In this niche of rhetorical activity, women are doing Internet research related to their own concern and returning to myPCOSteam to share their learning evidenced through examples of sharing information related to behavior and also products to alleviate symptoms.

One of the best examples of a myPCOSteam user engaging in self-research is Emilia15's post related to sleep apnea. Emilia15 first unpacks her history with sleep apnea, explaining how, one night, snoring from her sleep apnea woke her husband and kept him awake. She expresses guilt, saying, "I feel responsible for his bad night's sleep." She reiterates, "I feel so bad about it." Emilia15 then claims that she has "done some reading" and has identified a few solutions to help with sleep apnea. She notes:

> the main solutions seem to be losing weight (which as we all know is easier said than done with PCOS), sleeping on your side—which I do anyway, humidifier in the bedroom or eucalyptus essential oil rubbed on your chest.

Emilia15 concludes her post by asking if others struggle with sleep apnea and if they have any "tips" to offer.

Similar examples of self-research include researching and sharing with myPCOS-team users the products "Fertility Smart" and "Pregnitude," facts about ovarian cysts, and information about losing weight by cutting out dairy from the diet. The various self-actions by women on the forum reveal their commitments to being active participants in their own health, as well as in the health of others. By disseminating knowledge about alternative treatments for PCOS symptoms and about specific side effects of PCOS, the women actively go outside the knowledge established by medical authorities. In these ways, the rhetorical strategies reflect the values of MGT, such as looking outside the "dominant" group for knowledge and information that makes up a culture—in this case, the PCOS culture. Additionally, as the examples of self-research show, the rhetoric of this forum is reciprocal and respectful, values mirrored in FCT. These characteristics may best be explained in terms of patient agency—how actions that a patient takes outside of a clinical encounter are used to respond to the unique rhetorical needs of the patient and to their community (Arduser, 2017; Siegel Finer, 2016). In short, women with PCOS unpack and then act to solicit and share knowledge for the sake of their own health and for the health of others within myPCOSteam.

Conclusion

While an expanding corpus of research exists surrounding online health communities and their offerings for those with chronic illness, such as those with arthritis (e.g., Willis, & Royne, 2017), breast cancer (e.g., Sandaunet, 2008), and diabetes (e.g., Ho, O'Connor, & Mulvaney, 2014), until now, little was known about their offerings for women with PCOS. This study fills this gap by exploring one online health community, myPCOSteam, and by examining the rhetorical strategies that myPCOSteam users employed. Findings resulting from this study contribute to ongoing conversations surrounding women's health challenges and advocacy, as located within medical rhetoric scholarship.

Some of the results of this study are consistent with those derived by other researchers exploring how digital health communities support their users. For example, Setoyama et al. (2011) also identified themes suggesting that individuals participating in an online health community use the forums to exchange advice and provide various insights to others interacting within the site. Additionally, van der Eijk et al. (2013) found that online health communities provide opportunities for users to share experiences and exchange knowledge within the digital space. Although not a salient finding in this study, van der Eijk et al. (2013) further found that "due to rapid advances in medical knowledge, many health professionals lack sufficient expertise to address the complex health care needs of chronic patients" (p. 1438). Select participant posts in this study appear to validate van der Eijk et al.'s (2013) finding; it appears that when physicians have insufficient knowledge about treating women with PCOS, some physicians deflect and redirect the conversation when engaging with PCOS patients and explain, if the patient "just lost weight," the patient "wouldn't have PCOS" (Loren_Lasher02). The consistencies across these studies verify the offerings of online health communities and partly reveal the dismissive behaviors of some physicians treating women with PCOS.

To date, there is no cure for PCOS, and, as illustrated through the words of participants, PCOS is a wildly complex syndrome to treat. The health condition is multifaceted, with a variety of internal and external symptoms that PCOS patients can exhibit. One symptom can cause another to emerge. For example, insulin resistance can induce weight gain, which can induce hirsutism. Menstrual irregularities can assist in the manifestation of cystic acne, which can bring about anxiety and depression. Physicians term this phenomenon as comorbidity—when one or more physiological symptoms simultaneously occur. I do not cite sources within this paragraph about the effects of PCOS because, as a woman living with the syndrome, I know all too well about its associated symptoms. I live and breathe my syndrome. My syndrome impacts every bite of food I take and everything I drink. It affects my social interactions and my cognitive functions. It affects how much hair I lose while washing, combing, and styling and how I feel in my clothes. PCOS affects every facet of my life. It is my greatest foe.

Similar to the women I have studied, I have often found myself wondering how to ease my PCOS symptoms. Because a cure does not exist for PCOS, I have often searched the Internet for alternative PCOS treatments. Like those I have studied, I have participated in PCOS support groups to ask about the experiences of other women dealing with the syndrome. My actions can be viewed as enacting rhetorical ingenuity. Rather than accepting my syndrome and the symptoms that overtake my body, I choose to pursue various means that allow me to gain information that can potentially be used to better my own health. I share my PCOS experiences to reveal my positionality and connection to this research topic. My own PCOS experiences move me to advocate for greater PCOS awareness and for more research on PCOS so that, one day, a cure for the syndrome can possibly be found.

Notes

1 MyPCOSteam is hosted by MyHealthTeams, the same social network platform that hosts MyLupusTeam of interest to Pengilly, this collection.
2 This project was exempted by the IRB at Indiana University of Pennsylvania. In an effort to generate theory about the unique rhetorical strategies employed by women with PCOS in myPCOSteam, I used random sampling. This method was selected to limit the amount of data I collected and remove bias from data selection. I used a random integer generator, random.org, to give me a set of 25 numbers between 1 and 863, the total number of posts within myPCOSteam's forum at the time of data collection. Because this current project does not intend to make claims regarding the representativeness of the myPCOSteam data, but rather intends to locate and explain the rhetorical strategies employed by women within myPCOSteam, 25 posts were collected.
3 Note that the privacy policy for myPCOSteam members does not preclude me from directly quoting posts; however, pseudonyms are used for users' handles. Users' original language use has been retained, including errors.

References

Ardener, E. (1975). "Belief and the problem of women." In S. Ardener (Ed.). *Perceiving women* (pp. 1–17). London: Dent.

Arduser, L. (2017). *Living chronic: Agency and expertise in the rhetoric of diabetes.* Columbus, OH: The Ohio State Press.

Barry, J.A., Kuczmierczyk, A.R., & Hardiman, P.J. (2011). "Anxiety and depression in polycystic ovary syndrome: A systematic review and meta-analysis." *Human Reproduction*, 26(9), 2442–2451.

Beemer, C. (2016). "From the margins of healthcare: De-mythicizing cancer online." *Peitho*, 19(1), 93–127.

Christians, C.G. (2005). "Ethics and politics in qualitative research." In N.K. Denzin & Y. S. Lincoln (Eds.). *The Sage handbook of qualitative research* (pp. 139–164). Thousand Oaks, CA: Sage.

De Hertogh, L. (2015). "Reinscribing a new normal: Pregnancy, disability, and Health 2.0 in the online natural birthing community." *Birth Without Fear. Ada: A Journal of Gender, New Media, and Technology*, 1(7).

Denzin, N.K. (1996). *Interpretive ethnography: Ethnographic practices for the 21st century.* Thousand Oaks, CA: Sage.

Dobransky, K., & Hargittai, E. (2012). "Inquiring minds acquiring wellness: Uses of online and offline sources for health information." *Health Communication*, 27(4), 331–343.

Fox, S. (2011). *The social life of health information, 2011: Social media in context.* Washington, DC. Retrieved from Pew Research Center: www.pewinternet.org/2011/05/12/social-media-in-context/

Ho, Y.X., O'Connor, B.H., & Mulvaney, S.A. (2014). "Features of online health communities for adolescents with Type I diabetes." *Western Journal of Nursing Research*, 36(9), 1183–1198.

Holladay, D. (2017). "Classified conversations: Psychiatry and tactical technical communication in online spaces." *Technical Communication Quarterly*, 26(1), 8–24.

Househ, M., Borycki, E., & Kushniruk, A. (2014). "Empowering patients through social media: The benefits and challenges." *Health Informatics*, 20(1), 50–58.

Kramarae, C. (2009). "Muted group theory." In S.W. Littlejohn & K.A. Foss (Eds.). *Encyclopedia of communication theory* (pp. 667–669). Thousand Oaks, CA: Sage.

Pitts, V. (2004). "Illness and Internet empowerment: Writing and reading breast cancer in cyberspace." *Illness and Medicine*, 8(1), 33–59.

Saldaña, J. (2009). *The coding manual for qualitative researchers*. Thousand Oaks, CA: Sage.

Sandaunet, A.G. (2008). "A space for suffering? Communicating breast cancer in an online self-help context." *Qualitative Health Research*, 18(12), 1631–1641.

Setoyama, Y., Yamazaki, Y., & Nakayama, K. (2011). Comparing support to breast cancer patients from online communities and face-to-face support groups. *Patient Education and Counseling*, 85(2), 95–100. Retrieved from https://doi.org/10.1016/j.pec.2010.11.008

Siegel Finer, B. (2016). "The rhetoric of previving: Blogging the breast cancer gene." *Rhetoric Review*, 35(2), 176–188.

Tesch, R. (1990). *Qualitative research: Analysis types and software tools*. Philadelphia, PA: RoutledgeFalmer.

van der Eijk, M., Faber, M.J., Aarts, J.W., Kremer, J.A., Munneke, M., & Bloem, B.R. (2013). "Using online health communities to deliver patient-centered care to people with chronic conditions." *Journal of Medical Internet Research*, 15(6),e115.

Willis, E., & Royne, M.B. (2017). "Online health communities and chronic disease self-management." *Health Communication*, 32(3), 269–278.

US Department of Health and Human Services. (2016). "Polycystic ovary syndrome (PCOS)." Retrieved from www.womenshealth.gov/files/documents/pcos-factsheet.pdf

Yoo, W., Namkoong, K., Choi, M., Shah, D.V., Tsang, S., Hong, Y., … Gustafson, D.H. (2014). "Giving and receiving emotional support online: Communication competence as a moderator of psychosocial benefits for women with breast cancer." *Computers in Human Behavior*, 30, 12–22.

4

RHETORICS OF EMPOWERMENT FOR MANAGING LUPUS PAIN

Patient-to-Patient Knowledge Sharing in Online Health Forums

Cynthia Pengilly

I have lived *with, alongside,* and *through* lupus for several years; I lost my own mother to lupus when she was only 38. Of the approximately 1.5 million people in the United States who have lupus, over 90% are women (Lupus Foundation of America, 2018); as a black woman, I am nearly three times more likely to *die from* the disease than a non–Hispanic white woman (Izmirily et al., 2017; Fernandez et al., 2005). I have met countless other women who have shared their personal stories of suffering and frustration as they try to make sense of their life and the disease. When I turned 37, just a few days ago (at the time of writing), I was more relieved than celebratory. I may be managing my lupus better than my mother was able to at this age, considering her late diagnosis (i.e., I'm not hospitalized and/or bedridden), but I still have a long journey ahead before reaching my own sense of understanding of how to live with lupus. I participate in online patient forums as a way to educate myself, regain some semblance of agency and control, and connect with others who share my plight.

The growing significance of online health communities and forums in advancing patient agency and empowering strategies for self-care has been discussed in coverage of diabetes (Arduser, 2017), psychiatric care (Holladay, 2017), and PCOS (McKinley, this collection). Online lupus communities offer practical strategies for managing lupus that are often missing from formal publications of biomedical discourse such as medical pamphlets, medical websites, and even activist organizations' articles written and/or approved by medical doctors. One example of such a strategy is the recommended use of dietary supplements, which are often used in conjunction with, rather than in lieu of, prescription medications—a practical and useful strategy seemingly overlooked in formal medical discourse that is shared by lupus forum members.

The purpose of this study is to draw attention to competing discourses within the lupus community and to the role that rhetorics of empowerment can play at the micro level in advancing individual women's health. While narratives of suffering and instances of patient-led doctoring are not uncommon in the age of Web 2.0, I argue that patient-to-patient sharing of knowledge is especially empowering for lupus patients, chronic illness sufferers whose symptoms are not easily treated using traditional, top-down medical practices. Also, lupus forum patients have managed to create their own sort of biopsychosocial model of healthcare, often stepping outside the boundaries of traditional practice, which is deserving of further study. Thus, this chapter extends the work on chronic illness (Arduser, 2017; Derkatch, 2016; Holladay, 2017) by highlighting connections between chronic illness and CAM treatment options as they exist within the online space of lupus patient forums. Furthermore, this study focuses on women's health due to the overall ratio of women lupus sufferers, estimated at 90 % (Lupus Foundation of America, 2018) and contributes to RHM scholarship by exploring the intersection of chronic illness and women's health rhetorics.

Arduser (2017) identifies the struggles of the growing number of people with chronic illnesses who are managing and controlling symptoms so that they have the least amount of impact on daily life activities. This means locating strategies for managing the more prevalent symptoms of the disease such as fatigue, lupus-induced arthritis, and/or photosensitivity (Cojocaru et. al., 2011). The management process is especially difficult since chronic illness manifests differently in each patient, ranging from mild annoyances to severe, debilitating ailments, which arguably interrupt many chronic patients from reaching empowerment in their individual illness journey.

This lack of patient agency exists because chronic illness patients are less likely to be provided with a treatment plan that is as clear, direct, and measurable as acute diseases, which further contributes to the frustration and prolonged suffering of the patient (Arduser, 2017; Keränen, 2014). Consider, for example, the narrative account of the journey of a liver transplant patient, an acute disease with clear steps of progression (Angeli, & Johnson-Sheehan, 2018, p. 1). Particularly noteworthy is that the patient and his family were provided with two significant tools to aid in the illness journey: 1) "The Liver Team," the patient's team of specialized medical personnel, their different duties, and information about who to call when issues arise; and 2) the "Liver Transplant Education Binder," intended to guide the family through each stage of the transplant procedure. As someone suffering from a chronic illness with no obvious and identifiable path forward, I was astonished by the seemingly straightforward process (though I do not discount the difficult nature of the journey) and equally amazed by the communal aspects of patient care involving the patient, family, and team of specialists.

This study reveals a number of intersecting and competing interests between medical and patient discourses. In the first part, I identify a number of rhetorical barriers to patient self-care on medical information websites: WebMD, Lupus.

Org, and the US DHHS OWH website. I demonstrate how a rhetoric of deterrent model is used by these websites to redirect lupus patients towards approved treatments (operating as a Burkean terministic screen), further aided by a lack of specific, purposeful, and useful information for patients. The second part of this study identifies the communal aspects of two online health forums— The Lupus Site and MyLupusTeam. I pay particular attention to how the communities encourage patient interaction and knowledge sharing, evoking the psychosocial aspects of community care. In the third and final section, I draw attention to the power of patient-to-patient knowledge sharing in managing chronic illness. I provide extended examples of patient discourse about the individualized approaches to supplement use, especially when combined with prescription medication, which reveals a more empowering, caring, and informative approach for patients, that is nonetheless cautionary. Finally, this particular part of the study reveals the ways that patient-to-patient communication can operate as sites of resistance to doctor-centered treatment plans while still encouraging a strong doctor-patient relationship.

Rhetorical Barriers to Patient Self-Care on Medical Websites

Medical websites play a large role in patient self-care, as even lupus patient forums link directly to sites such as WebMD, Lupus Foundation, and the OWH. Arguably, this is especially the case with chronic illnesses since the patient must become knowledgeable about how the illness operates both inside and outside the boundaries of biomedicine; in other words, chronic illness patients must learn to navigate their everyday lives alongside the illness (Arduser, 2017; Derkatch, 2016). For instance, the rhetoric of medical discourse encourages diabetes patients to become "experts" on their condition and "informed consumers" with regard to medical technology, thus elevating the status of medical literature in the patient's day-to-day life (Arduser, 2017). This medical practice is also repeated for lupus patients, who are similarly encouraged to manage their condition, but with considerably less specificity.

The primary treatment advice provided to lupus patients, for example, is often narrowly limited to monitoring diet, exercise, stress, and sleep (US DHHS, 2017b; 2018). The generality of such a treatment plan is likely because lupus is difficult to diagnose, treat, and manage; it manifests itself differently in each patient, one of the few consistently acknowledged aspects of the disease. However, such recommendations are too general to be useful to patients seeking knowledge about the inner workings of the disease (i.e., big picture) and everyday practical strategies for managing the disease (i.e., little picture). For example, in the "Lupus and Women Fact Sheet" (US DHHS, 2017a), patients are given the following information in the opening paragraph: "There is no cure for lupus, but treatments can help you feel better and improve your symptoms." However, treatment options are minimally addressed and buried within the section titled, "What can I do to *control* my symptoms?" (emphasis my own) alongside options used to control and manage the illness (diet, stress, exercise, etc.). Surprisingly, only one line is directly related to treatment: "Taking medicines to reduce swelling and pain, calm your immune system, and reduce damage to the joints or organs," but it fails to identify the most common medications used by lupus patients to achieve these outcomes, thereby reducing its usefulness for patients. In a longer explanation on the OWH website, the section, "Controlling My Lupus," expands to include "following your treatment plan" and "see your doctors regularly" (US DHHS, 2018). In this section, three direct references to seeking a doctor's assistance are made as well as three indirect references—i.e., make a treatment plan, set realistic goals, and build a support system of people you trust. Similar language and tactics are found within WebMD as well, which limit patient decision-making and force patients back into the biomedical model of doctor-controlled care.

The rhetorical barriers to alternative treatment options can also be found in the discourses surrounding supplements on medical websites. On the OWH site, for instance, patients are provided with a list of six categories of medicines for treating lupus: NSAIDs, corticosteroids, antimalarials, BLys-specific inhibitors, immunosuppressive drugs, and "other" medicines. The category of "other" does not mention supplements or alternative medicines, suggesting that these are still regarded as "quackery" in medical discourse (Derkatch, 2016), even though supplements are used by more than half of all adults in the US, as reported by the CDC on WedMD (Afshar, 2015). Instead, supplements are discussed as an appended item toward the end of the section under the "Talk to Your Doctor" heading, followed by a list of cautionary items or special circumstances, such as side effects, new symptoms, and pregnancy.

This practice is not too dissimilar from "caution" or "notes" elements in technical and professional writing documents, meant to discourage readers from continuing the search or otherwise straying from the "right" path. In this case, the right path is biomedicine, which does not openly support the use of supplements.

Similar language is found on WebMD and the Lupus Foundation websites with regard to supplement use by patients experiencing joint pain. This language discourages patient empowerment in two significant ways: 1) by employing a rhetoric of doubt as a warning against the use of supplements; and 2) by employing a rhetoric of deterrence by providing few practical strategies for the use of supplements. The first notable example is a WebMD article (Afshar, 2015) that begins by acknowledging the growing use of supplements across the world and in the US: "People in some parts of the world have used herbal remedies to treat diseases for centuries … A 2011 survey from the CDC found that more than half of all adults in the US take one of these products." It simultaneously admits its lack of acceptance in the US: "we tend to rely heavily on traditional Western medicine." These two paragraphs serve as soft openers, rhetorically speaking, to the blow that is to come regarding the use of supplements due to lack of verifiable evidence.

The WebMD article continues by identifying several popular herbal remedies to treat joint pain (e.g., fish oil, borage oil, boswellia, ginger, green tea,
and probiotics), but also shrouding them in a rhetoric of doubt due to either
reported side-effects or the lack of scientific studies conducted by the medical
community. The rhetoric of doubt is also employed on several Lupus.org
pages with regard to the use of supplements. Here is one such example:
"Most alternative and complementary practices, however, have not been
through the rigorous scientific testing and clinical research that all conventional medicines undergo, so it is difficult to know their effectiveness in
treating lupus" (Lupus Foundation of America, 2013b). The primary means of
rigorous, scientific testing noted here is RCT testing, a scientific methodology
and evidence-gathering process, which concludes that traditional biomedicine
itself often does not meet stringent RCT standards (Derkatch, 2016). Instead,
RCT is an ideal standard of biomedicine to be used in an ideal environment
with ideal patients, which is impossible to obtain. Derkatch (2016) identifies
instances when biomedicine is not held to the same standards as CAM, a fact
only privy to those in the medical community, thereby limiting the rhetorical
agency of patients. As such, the RCT gold standard has taken on the role of
gatekeeper for any new, innovative medical treatments, such as the use
of supplements. When taken together, the medical discourse operates as a set of
terministic screens or language designed to direct an audience toward a particular
perception (Burke, 1966); in this case, biomedical discourse of these websites,
with their rhetoric of doubt, leads patients towards a particular conclusion (i.e.,
supplements are inferior forms of medicine and are dangerous).

The irony of warnings about herbal supplements is that the side effects listed
are similar to some of the medicines approved for lupus pain; in some cases,
supplements can have fewer side effects. Take Plaquenil—the leading prescription
used by lupus patients to alleviate joint pain, swelling, skin rashes, and fatigue;
side effects are well known to include itching/hives, stomach pain, blisters, vision
deterioration, nausea, vomiting, and headaches, among others. The side effects of
vision deterioration, specifically retinal damage, appears frequently as a topic in
lupus patient forums, ranging from general comments ("be sure to check your
vision each year") to explicit warnings against the medication ("vision is so bad I
cannot drive myself to work anymore"). Alternative treatments for joint pain
include fish oil, turmeric, boswellia, and barrage oil. Boswellia, for example,
which has been through medical testing with "mixed findings" (Afshar, 2015),
has the same level of pain relief as NSAIDs, such as ibuprofen. And, while it does
have side effects such as diarrhea, nausea, and rash if applied directly to the skin,
boswellia does not have the associated stomach problems noted with NSAIDs.
The reality of supplement use and its related side effects for managing lupus differ
quite a bit from the medical discourse surrounding it; the terministic screen
employed through the rhetoric of doubt continues to reinforce biomedical practices. Along those same lines, Derkatch (2016) posits that while the boundaries of

biomedicine may have expanded slightly to include aspects of CAM, such as acupuncture and dietary supplements, biomedicine has mostly kept its doctor-centered model of care and methods of evidence intact so as not to weaken its authority and legitimacy in the medical community. As a result, in the case of lupus patients, medical discourse has the potential to act as a rhetorical deterrent rather than a rhetoric of empowerment.

This rhetorical deterrent model is also evident in the limited practical information. On WebMD, for example, even when herbal remedies such as bowel-lisa and probiotics are noted to have the potential to relieve pain, patients are provided with only a few sentences of information. Furthermore, the various hyperlinked phrases link patients to a page about the supplement where it is discussed as a broad category (e.g., "holistic medicine") without specific and targeted uses of the supplement for those suffering from joint pain or arthritis. This model is similarly employed on Lupus.org, where patients are presented with a list of CAM treatment options, although few are hyperlinked to even broad additional information. Patients must leave the page to search the terms on their own if they hope to explore alternative care options.

The Lupus Foundation page does include one hyperlink to the National Center for Complementary and Integrative Health located at the very end of the page. While this resource may be useful, the link does not take patients to the page, or group of pages, specifically dealing with lupus-related care. This practice distances patients from the essential knowledge needed to gain agency and control over the illness in a manner that best fits their desires. The rhetoric of doubt combined with the limited practical information on supplemental medicines serve as deterrents, since even just the knowledge of supplements or possession of more well-rounded understanding of alternative medicines can be empowering, even if the patient declines to participate.

The collective rhetoric of the medical community might appear to be in favor of increasing patient agency on the surface, but the actual practices and discourses shifts authority back to biomedical standards, reinforcing the power dynamics most common to the biomedical model of care. The lupus medical community may also be unwittingly limiting—rather than aiding—women's knowledge and agency in reaching a deeper understanding of their own health and healthcare. This is, however, somewhat mitigated by the knowledge work taking place in online patient forums.

Communal Aspects of Online Health Forums

The previous section analyzed medical websites to reveal rhetorics of doubt and deterrence. I posit, in similar fashion to Derkatch (2016), that such rhetorical and philosophical underpinnings are not always a conscious attempt by the medical community to restrict patient agency, since rhetorical persuasion can be both conscious and unconscious. However, the response by patients to participate in online lupus forums—whether for general guidance, a sense of community, or active displays of resistance—is indeed conscious. I turn to patient rhetoric and knowledge sharing in this section as a direct response to medical discourse.

As a lupus patient, I became a member of The Lupus Site[1] and MyLupusTeam in my illness journey while seeking understanding and practical management of my own condition, from where I've drawn the excerpts in this chapter.[2] Patients shape their own cultures in online forums—a shared concept of illness within a particular medical sub-group—and this culture has *communal identification*, which "along with each venue's relative privacy, leads to candid conversations about experiences with social and psychological distress, behavioral differences, and medical interventions" (Holladay, 2017, p. 8). The actions of forum participants are invisible to biomedical institutions and organizations that are chiefly concerned with acute disease and how to control it, as opposed to chronic illness, which is uncontrollable and unpredictable (Holladay, 2017).

The patient forums are organized in such a manner as to encourage patient-to-patient knowledge sharing in general, as members are presented with a number of options for self-learning or interaction, including but not limited to links to fact sheets, practical information, and community, where the forum and member list is located. Within the forum itself, users can like a post, follow a thread, and link to other users' posts. The Lupus Site's architecture and forum capabilities date back to 1997, the first year of its copyright, but the interactive options for posts are more contemporary in nature since users can endorse a post with such labels as: I recommend, I suggest, I like/liked, I agree, I pray/prayers/prayed. The lengthy history of this site speaks to the demand for community-driven healthcare sites that extend beyond the purview of the biomedical hierarchy.

MyLupusTeam brands itself as "a social network for those living with lupus," and it features a number of different options for socialization. Profile pages can be updated with a story or illness journey, list of treatments, "MyLupusTeam" members (a combination of other MyLupusTeam site users, non-profit organizations, and/or local doctors), recommendations, a question-answer area, pinboards for photo sharing, and favorites. These are some of the many ways the forum blends biomedical and psychosocial aspects together as a working unit. There are also several options within the forum to encourage interaction (see Figure 4.1). Members can give a hug, mark a post as useful, mention users directly in a post, add a member to their personal lupus team, add a post to favorites, and set a lupus status of the day (good, bad, so/so).

Figure 4.1 shows my status update with the "so/so" tag; I received several "hugs" from other members in a matter of minutes. When writing, I experience a lupus flare due to stress associated with the task of writing itself and the anxiety of the looming deadline; I am always writing *alongside* and *within* the midst of illness. In the case of this chapter, I struggled to find separation between myself, my illness, and my writing—indeed, the very definition of meta self-awareness—a point I commiserated about with my fellow lupus community. Generally speaking, social support is understood to be a positive coping mechanism for chronic

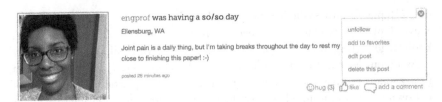

FIGURE 4.1 Post Page on MyLupusTeam

illness patients, resulting in less anxiety and stress (Holladay, 2017; Arduser, 2017), which happen to be triggers for lupus flares (Lupus Foundation of America, 2013a). Thus, these preliminary findings of the bio + psychosocial elements of lupus patient forums suggest that these spaces function as encouraging and safe spaces for a number of different patient-to-patient activities.

Patient-to-Patient Knowledge Sharing

One noteworthy example of patient-to-patient knowledge sharing that makes strong rhetorical moves toward patient agency and empowerment is the discussion surrounding supplements. Current medical practice is to treat lupus pain first by NSAIDs and/or opioids, followed by corticosteroids, antimalarials, and immune suppressants (Criscione-Schreiber, 2017). A similar treatment procedure is also recommended on WebMD and the Lupus Foundation, with fewer than 1% of site pages devoted to the discussion of supplements or CAM. Alternatively, more diverse strategies are discussed on the lupus patient forums, where patients freely share their lists of medications and information on drug trials and recent medical studies. On The Lupus Site, for instance, supplements exist in approximately 20% of forum topics with titles such as: "Supplements that I take," "Request for Advice on Supplements," "What supplements do you take with your daily regime?" Supplements are discussed frequently in patient forums, a trend that is clearly overlooked by medical discourse.

One pattern that emerged was the combination of prescription medications and supplements. Online patient discourse contains exchanges on *why* supplements can be useful to lupus patients and strategies on *how* to combine supplements with other treatment options. The following patient exchanges are drawn from the thread titled, "Supplements I find that help ..." from The Lupus Site (emphasis my own):

PATIENT 1: After not knowing what was wrong with me for such a long time i finally got to see [doctor name removed] who *suggested* taking Gingko Biloba tablets which i started straight away since then I've added the following: Ginsing, Omega 3 fish oils (not fish liver oils), Multi Vitamins, Evening Primrose Oil, Epervestant Vitamin C. These are taken along side my *daily prescribed medication* & i am wanting to find out if there's anything else anyone can suggest as it is I'm taking 13 tablets on a morning alone. After starting the supplements i have found i am feeling so much better & didn't catch the horrible cold my other half had which I'd usually do as I've no immune system after having a full splenectomy due to ITP caused by SLE :/

This excerpt is promising for other lupus patients on the forum who might be interested in alternative care models, as the patient reveals two important elements: 1) the patient found a doctor amenable to dietary supplements to aid in lupus management; and 2) the doctor is willing to recommend a *specific* supplement. The patient, as a newcomer to the lupus community, is likely unaware of the uniqueness of her doctor–patient relationship, as she glosses over these two important aspects in a single opening clause ("i finally got to see [doctor name removed] who suggested taking Gingko Biloba"). However, her combination of prescription and supplements in her lupus treatment plan follows a trend in the lupus community forums, which encourages other responses in kind.

For instance, Patient 2's response is specific in terms of the medication plan; she noticeably lingers on patient–doctor communication and weighing the advice of others, most likely due to Patient 1's status as a novice, both to the illness itself and the online lupus community. See the two excerpts below (emphasis my own):

PATIENT 2: Over the past three years, I've been given TONS of advice from people who either have lupus or know someone who does. I've taken their advice and discussed the options with my rheumy. Here's what I take on a daily basis: In the *early afternoon*, I take 2 tablets Calcium 600 mg, 2 tablets Glucosamine Chondroitin, 1 tablet Stress B Complex, 1 capsule Turmeric Curcumin, 1 gel Vitamin A 8000 iu and 1 gel Vitamin D 5000 iu. *At night* I take another 2 tablets of Glucosamine Chondroitin, and another turmeric curcumin. I also take 1 tablet Magnesium, 1 tablet Potassium along with 20 mg Omeprazole and 200 mg Plaquenil. *Every three days*, I take an iron pill. I fully believe this regimen has kept me from being in pain and unable to do what I do on a daily basis. But I also know that [what] may be good for one person may not produce the same results with someone else. Take my suggestions, consult with your Rheumatologist and/or your Primary and use their medical knowledge to guide you.

In this lengthy response, Patient 2 shares her illness experience and provides great detail about her medication plan, all while demonstrating great care in her response. First, she encourages a strong patient–doctor dialogue about managing the individual illness journey: "discussed the options with my rheumy" and "Take my suggestions, consult with your Rheumatologist and/or your Primary and use their medical knowledge to guide you." The patient accepted advice from others prior to adding supplements to her treatment plan: "Over the past three years, I've been given TONS of advice from people who either have lupus or know someone who does," which served as a rhetoric of empowerment in guiding her own illness journey. Next, Patient 2 provides specific information about how primary and supplemental medicines can be used together in managing daily lupus pain, identifying "early afternoon" medications, which are all supplements, including the iron pill, and night time medications, more supplements and Plaquenil, the only prescription medication.

After receiving the response from Patient 2, which strongly encourages open doctor–patient communication, Patient 1 replies with additional clarification on her medications and reiterates that her treatment plan has been approved by her doctor. Other patients chime in with shorter responses (i.e., listing one supplement without mention of how it was selected and/or if it is taken in conjunction with a prescription med), which fits a larger pattern across both lupus websites— short discussions of individualized treatment plans involving supplements scattered throughout the entire site, rather than grouped in a single location.

Such hesitation on the part of lupus patients could be a reflection of biomedicine's successful boundary-work (Derkatch, 2016), making some patients reluctant to openly discuss supplements for fear of ridicule; after all, even the medical discourse on lupus websites reinforces this stereotype, as previously discussed. This could be subconscious, especially if looking at individual patients operating solely in the biomedical model of care; however, the very nature of online forums encourages patients to expand their understanding of everyday life, and by extension, their understanding of illness. As Holladay (2017) points out, actions of forum participants are (theoretically) invisible to institutions and organizations that would impose order, which allows them to use the forum to bridge their diagnosis with everyday lived experiences. Patients are encouraged to explore the unimaginable in a safe space where others like them have also pondered on, or participated in, the same activities. In this way, the communal aspect of the site serves as a place of resistance to the biomedical model and infrastructure, which operates on a conscious level. With this in mind, the lack of a site-wide discussion on supplements can be interpreted as being aligned with other CAM practices due to the nature of individualized, patient-centered treatments in CAM.

Take, for example, this second exchange between two patients on MyLupusTeam. Other members of the community can see the posts, but do not comment. As a community, we can provide guidance to one another based only on what has worked at the individual level.

PATIENT 3: Hi [name removed], I just started to try the Functional Medicine. I am seeing a dietitian, who used Functional Medicine to treat her own MS. Could you share the protocol you used? What food have you eliminated from your diet? What supplements are you taking? How long had you been on it before you started to see improvements? Thank you!

PATIENT 4: Sure I'm happy to share! I went on a very strict elimination diet where I basically ate only fruit, veggies (no nightshades), fish, chicken (organic) and grass fed beef, and rice. This was for 6 weeks then I gradually added in items one by one and looked for reactions ... I am taking 4.5 mg of Low Dose Naltrexone each night as well as the following each day. Vit C, D3, A, B multi, DHEA 25mg, CurcuPlex-95, a probiotic, a prebiotic and a digestive enzyme (SoectraZyme Metagest). I started having a marked reduction in pain 4 weeks into the elimination diet ... I've also been meditating regularly for 19 days and that is helping with stress (which also brings on pain) a lot. Check out Dr Connie Jeon online—Lupus Rebel. She has a ton of good info too for a small subscription fee.

PATIENT 3: (follow-up): Thank you so much for the detailed info. I found that it is really hard to find the right diet ... There are Vegan diet, Paleo diet, and Pagan diet. ... I believe that diet can help with managing lupus. I just don't know what to follow. I started with an all plant based vegan diet. I felt that it help with the joint pain. But I thought I was not getting enough protein and maybe other nutrition as well, such as B12. I started to see a dietitian ... So, I added fish and lean chicken meat to my diet and removed gluten ... I started to take probiotics too, and I will start with the milti-vitamin next week. We will see what happens. I will definitely check out Dr Connie Jeon. Did you book an appointment with her? I am glad that you figured out what the foods you had reactions to. I find this is the hardest part of this process. Was it easy for you to figure it out? Do you have any tips on how you figured it out? Thanks!

[This exchange continues as each patient answers questions from the previous post, often including more strategies, and concludes with recommendations (in the case of Patient 4) or additional questions (in the case of Patient 3).]

Ultimately, the two lupus patients share a common belief—diet helps with managing lupus—and they use the forum to help them achieve a common goal: Establishing the right diet for their specific type of lupus and their specific bodily responses to food. The process is complicated, but as the exchanges grow in length and specificity, it is clear that the process is working; these women are engaging in a level of patient-to-patient knowledge sharing beyond the boundaries of biomedicine. In this communal space, patients are able to translate vague medical information provided to all lupus patients into practical knowledge on the connections and intersections between diet, medications, and illness.

This narrative exchange demonstrates, along with scattered discussions of supplements across both lupus sites, that the decision to include supplements in lupus pain management need not be an either/or dichotomy. In fact, the use of supplements is but one aspect of a multifaceted approach to lupus care that is only hinted at in the medical discourse. Furthermore, the examples presented here also speak to the biopsychosocial aspects of community care already embedded in the daily activities of online health forums.

Conclusion

Patient agency is a highly contested concept in a new world of patient-centered healthcare. As identified by several scholars in RHM, the medical community has been tasked with addressing the growth of chronic illnesses through the design and development of new patient-centered care models that include increased opportunity for shared decision-making practices (Arduser, 2017; Derkatch, 2016), where chronic care patients must be active communicators with an interest in "sharing knowledge as well as producing knowledge" (Arduser, 2017, p. 6). However, what Arduser (2017) and Derkatch (2016) highlight is the lack of doctor–patient collaboration and the various types and levels of restriction placed on patients in managing their own self-care. Patient compliance is still underlying the collaborative patient model.

The preliminary findings in this study suggest that the bio + psychosocial elements of lupus patient forums have the potential to help chronic illness patients regain agency by re-situating the patient-centered care model to one that is equally individual and community-driven. Because lupus manifests itself differently in every woman, it makes pattern recognition difficult to track on a macro level (across medical discourse) but perhaps easier to pinpoint on a micro level (between patients), which is why patient-to-patient interaction is so essential to patient agency and the successful management of chronic illness. Online forum patients routinely work against biomedical standardizations of care and revise medical advice to reflect their own illness experience or journey (Holladay, 2017). Holladay draws a distinction between biomedical strategies, which have obvious limitations (controlling acute disease), and patient tactics, which are tied to everyday lived experiences of illness. The rhetorical moves that lupus patients use to empower themselves and others with tested solutions, despite the constraining medical community pressures, demonstrate the potential for patient forums to operate as sites of resistance to traditional biomedical practice and sites of empowerment for the type of patient-centered care advocated by Arduser (2017) and Derkatch (2016).

I have only just begun my own illness journey, but I feel empowered through my own interactions in the forums and by observing the various points of interaction between others, each of whom exist at different stages along the illness journey continuum. Within the forums, a patient has the opportunity to engage with others or simply to read the information presented as a silent participant, to acquire the necessary depth and breadth of knowledge for navigating her own illness journey in the future. Both options are a form of patient interaction and knowledge sharing that afford opportunities for patient empowerment.

Notes

1 Note MyLupusTeam is hosted by MyHealthTeams, the same social network platform that hosts MyPCOSteam of interest to McKinley, this collection.
2 Note that the privacy policy for The Lupus Site and MyLupusTeam members does not preclude me from directly quoting posts; however, I do anonymize users' names and handles. Users' original language use has been retained, including errors.

References

Afshar, B. (2015). "11 herbs and supplements for rheumatoid arthritis to take or avoid." Retrieved from: www.webmd.com/rheumatoid-arthritis/features/rheumatoid-arthritis-best-worst-supplements-herbs#2

Angeli, E.L., & Johnson-Sheehan, R. (2018). "Introduction to the special issue: Medical humanities and/or the rhetoric of health and medicine." *Technical Communication Quarterly*, 27(1), 1–6.

Arduser, L. (2017). *Living chronic: Agency and expertise in the rhetoric of diabetes*. Columbus, OH: Ohio State University Press.

Burke, K. (1966). "Terministic Screens." *Language as symbolic action: Essays on life, literature, and method*. Berkeley, CA: University of California Press.

Cojocaru, M., Cojocaru, I.M., Silosi, I., & Vrabie, C.D. (2011). "Manifestations of systemic lupus erythematosus." *Maedica: A Journal of Clinical Medicine*, 6(4): 330–336.

Criscione-Schreiber, L. (2017). "Managing pain in active or well-controlled systemic lupus erythematosus." *Practical Pain Management*, 12(1). Retrieved from www.practicalpainmanagement.com/pain/myofascial/autoimmune/managing-pain-active-well-controlled-systemic-lupus-erythematosus

Derkatch, C. (2016). *Bounding biomedicine: Evidence and rhetoric in the new science of alternative medicine*. Chicago, IL: University of Chicago Press.

Fernandez, M., Calvo-Alen, J., Alarcon, G.S., et al. (2005). "Systemic lupus erythematosus in a multiethnic US cohort (LUMINA): XXI. Disease activity, damage accrual, and vascular events in pre- and postmenopausal women." *Arthritis Rheum*, 52(6), 1655–1664.

Holladay, D. (2017). "Classified conversations: Psychiatry and tactical technical communication in online spaces." *Technical Communication Quarterly*, 26(1), 8–24.

Izmirly, P.M., WanI., SahlS., BuyonJ.P., BelmontH.M., SalmonJ.E., ... PartonH. (2017). "The incidence and prevalence of systemic lupus erythematosus in New York County (Manhattan), New York: The Manhattan lupus surveillance program." *Arthritis Rheumatol*, 69(10), 2006–2017.

Keränen, L. (2014). "'This weird, incurable disease': Competing diagnoses in the rhetoric of morgellons." In T. Jones, L. Friedman, & D. Wear (Eds.), *Health humanities reader* (pp. 36–49). New Brunswick, NJ: Rutgers University Press.

Lupus Foundation of America. (2013a). "Common triggers for lupus." Retrieved from https://resources.lupus.org/entry/common-triggers

Lupus Foundation of America. (2013b). "Are there complementary and alternative medicine therapies for lupus?" Retrieved from https://resources.lupus.org/entry/complementary-and-alternative-medicines

Lupus Foundation of America. (2018). "Lupus Facts and Statistics." Retrieved from https://resources.lupus.org/entry/facts-and-statistics

US Department of Health and Human Services. (2017a). "Lupus and women." Fact sheet. Retrieved from www.womenshealth.gov/files/documents/fact-sheet-lupus.pdf

US Department of Health and Human Services. (2017b). "Lupus fact sheet." Retrieved from www.lb7.uscourts.gov/documents/13cv43867.pdf

US Department of Health and Human Services. (2018). "Living with lupus." Retrieved from www.womenshealth.gov/lupus/living-lupus

5

RHETORICS OF SELF-DISCLOSURE

A Feminist Framework for Infertility Activism

Maria Novotny and Lori Beth De Hertogh

It's late summer, the time of year when I clean out my closets in an effort to physically and mentally switch from the relaxed spirit of summer to the bustle of fall classes. I reach for the closet's top shelf, grabbing for a small pile of empty boxes I meant to throw away months ago. Instead of hard cardboard edges, my hand touches something soft, tender. It's a teddy bear with brown eyes and a bright red scarf. A teddy bear my brother gave to me long ago. A teddy bear I've kept with the thought that I might one day gently place it in a baby's crib. I feel my chest tighten: Do I leave the teddy bear in the closet? Do I give it to our puppy (my new "furbaby") as a toy? Do I keep it with the hope that, despite years of failure, I might still become pregnant?

Lori Beth

As I begin to draft my dissertation, I sit perched in the room that was to be the baby's. I am rereading some infertility narratives that I collected for my research when I become overwhelmed by memories. Momentary bits of sadness roll over me like a fog. I recall when my husband and I first purchased this home and imagined this bedroom as our future nursery. Where my desk sits is where we had hoped a crib would rest. Recalling the excitement we once had for our future, I am suddenly awoken by our dog's bark. The fog of sadness breaks, and I realize how much I have changed over the last five years. My infertility has changed me, and writing about infertility has changed me. Meeting other infertile women, hearing their stories, honoring them in my dissertation—I am grateful for who I have now become: a storyteller. I write stories of reproductive loss to make space for the grief I, along with millions of other women, have too long suffered in silence.

Maria

Introduction

The above stories illustrate the core premise informing this chapter: Infertility activism begins with self-disclosure. Our decision to draw the reader's attention to our infertile bodies is intentional and models how we see health activism as an embodied experience, particularly within the context of infertility. In fact, the exigence for this chapter began when we (the authors) shared our own infertility stories with each other. This would happen as we quietly talked in a corner of a conference center or via direct messages on Twitter. Yet these disclosures were always conducted in private. This led us to ask: Why are such disclosures often limited to private spaces, and how might this chapter and, indeed, this edited collection help us shift these conversations to more public forums?

We argue in this chapter that self-disclosure, or what we call *rhetorics of self-disclosure*, is a critical component of infertility activism. Social norms and discourses that link experiences of "womanhood" to those of "motherhood" pressure individuals of all backgrounds, ethnicities, and races to keep narratives of infertility cloistered within the private sphere (Ulrich, & Weatherall, 2000). Further, because of advancements in fertility treatment, many infertile individuals opt to privately undergo treatment and avoid self-disclosure (Bute, 2013). Yet, there are many psychosocial health issues that can emerge due to the rhetorical silencing of infertility (Allison, 2011). For example, mental health clinicians working with infertile patients cite a range of psychological stressors, including the financial out-of-pocket costs for alternative family-building (such as adoption or invitro fertilization), the experience of undergoing fertility treatment, and increased marital distress (Cousineau,& Domar, 2007). Such pressures are even greater for men and women of color whose infertility experiences are also mediated by race. Racial stereotypes of African American women, for instance, portray them "as having unusual stamina, independence, and perseverance" that uniquely suits them to motherhood (Ceballo, Graham, & Hart, 2015, p. 505). Such stereotyping can pressure African American women to "remain silent about reproductive problems because they believe they should be able to handle these difficulties alone, as strong self-reliant women" (pp. 504–505). In short, silence has a real, embodied impact on the health of the infertile body.

To demonstrate how rhetorics of self-disclosure inform health activism, we explain how cultural narratives of pregnancy unintentionally silence narratives of reproductive loss and how self-disclosing infertility acts as a counterstory to such narratives. Next, we build on the work of scholars such as Arola (2014), Vinson (2017), Novotny (2019), and Johnson and Quinlan (2017) to argue that rhetorics of self-disclosure are an essential component of infertility activism. To demonstrate how rhetorics of self-disclosure can transform conversations around infertility, we draw from our own embodied experiences of infertility and from the work of advocacy organizations such as RESOLVE: The National Infertility Association. We conclude by discussing the limitations and affordances of self-disclosure as a feminist, health activist framework.

Celebrating Pregnancy, Closeting Infertility

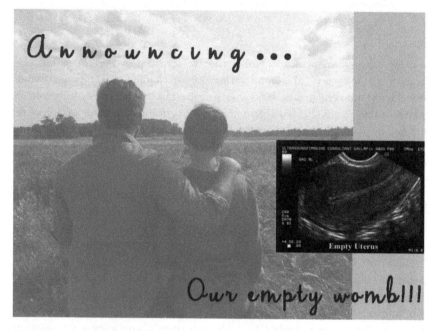

FIGURE 5.1 Mock Announcement

I created this "mock" announcement in a visual rhetoric graduate course. At the time, I was coming to terms with my infertility diagnosis. Tired and frustrated by what seemed like daily pregnancy announcements, I became angry that I would most likely never share such an announcement. Thinking about this, I realized that I did have something to announce: my infertility. I decided to make my own postcard sized "mock" announcement to reflect the loneliness my partner and I felt as friends and family members shared with us their news of a growing family. After making this piece, I wondered how others would react if I actually sent it to them or shared it on Facebook. Would they feel the same pain and loneliness I do? Would this postcard make them think twice about how lucky they are to be able to get pregnant naturally? "Probably not," I thought to myself.

Maria

In 2012, I began working with an online childbirth community that would become my primary research site for the next six years. When I first became involved with this community, I had no idea I was infertile, and I enjoyed learning about pregnancy and childbirth from community members and in turn imagining what my own childbirth experience might be like. But as time went on and I "failed" to become pregnant, my relationship with the community—and my own academic identity—changed. I began to feel like a phony, an imposter, a fake; like

I didn't have a right to do pregnancy research because I could not carry a child. When I presented my research at conferences or shared it with colleagues, I never publicly revealed that I was infertile; I preferred for people to that think I was one of those ambitious academics who was just waiting for the "right time" to have kids.

Lori Beth

In many cultures, pregnancy and childbirth are occasions that call for public celebration. Couples post ultrasound images on social media; family and friends attend baby showers; grandparents display baby photos on desks, walls, and in holiday cards. Arola (2014) suggests that these actions are a form of epideictic rhetoric, or public rhetorics of ceremony and celebration. Aristotle combined the concepts of public praise and *epideixis* as the rhetorical concept *encomium*, a form of public rhetoric intended to honor and praise a particular person, event, or cultural value (Pernot, 2015, p. 5).

Encomium is useful for considering the ways pro-natalist societies culturally and rhetorically re-inscribe fertility as a state of being worthy of public recognition, celebration, and praise. Discourses of infertility, by contrast, are silenced, circulating almost exclusively within the private sphere. Arola (2011) contends that narratives of infertility "remain silent" and are removed from our public "life narrative" because "we are not comfortable with infertility." Despite the 12% of women and about 8% of men in the US who experience what the CDC (2016) calls "impaired fecundity," public disclosures of infertility seem to trouble their audiences. For instance, Arola (2011) observes that "if you answer the question 'any kids?' with 'no, I'm infertile,' you can watch the asker's face cringe with regret; they wish you remained silent, they wish your rhetorical act is one of avoidance, of implicitly agreeing with our current notions of family."

The idea that infertility should remain silent or limited to private conversations within the domestic or medical sphere can be traced to historical notions of propriety and fertility. Jensen (2015), for example, notes that 19th-century notions of fertility were rooted in the view that the reproductive aspects of a woman's body are machine-like "parts" that need to be "fixed" in order to properly operate (pp. 27–36). This approach situated a woman's reproductive features into two categories: If the female reproductive system was "broken" (i.e., infertile), then discourses around the body should be limited to the home or medical sphere until the situation could be remedied (i.e., a woman became pregnant). By contrast, evidence that a woman's reproductive system was "working" (i.e., pregnancy) shifted conversations around reproduction from the domestic to the public sphere, where a women's fertility could be openly disclosed and celebrated.

Jensen's work offers historical perspective on infertility and how it is rhetorically constructed as a private matter: "it is difficult not to draw parallels between these discourses of the past and discourses of the present day" (p. 42). For example, our own narratives reveal how publicly disclosing one's infertility remains fraught with social, personal, and professional difficulties. In other words, the rhetorical frameworks of the past that silenced infertility and relegated it to the private sphere remain firmly in place today.

Silencing, we argue, is not just a discursive act; it is also embodied. Some bodies can remain silent as they have no physical "outed" attributes, while others carry signifiers that make them visible to others. This is because "the body also carries *signifying power*, articulating some of any body's many affiliations (Johnson et al., 2015, p. 40). For example, a pregnant body can hide only briefly. Frost and Haas (2017) elaborate on the rhetorical visibility of pregnant bodies in their decolonial critique of fetal ultrasounds: "[many individuals] privilege observation of what is made visible by the ultrasound procedure, the real-time ultrasound images, and the take-home sonogram image to distribute as evidence of our bodies' fertility potential" (p. 93). The visual artifact, the sonogram, evidences one's fertility and evokes public celebration. Yet for bodies that undergo an ultrasound and discover no pregnancy, and perhaps, even fertility issues—the sonogram is not distributed or shared, as demonstrated by Maria's mock announcement.

Rhetorics of Self-Disclosure: An Embodied Framework for Feminist Health Activism

Self-disclosure is a feminist rhetorical practice that contemplatively "tacks in" to moments when infertile bodies are perceived as invisible or erased (Royster, & Kirsch, 2012). When women self-disclose and make their experiences of infertility visible to others, they become "agents in the process" of feminist rhetorical action (p. 86) and, we add, activism. Yet, self-disclosing infertility—when situated as a personal, intimate, and private experience—can leave one in a vulnerable position. Uthappa (2017) writes "to fight stigma through narratives of self-disclosure, the speaker and the audience member's willingness to take a vulnerable stance—to grant potentially change-producing agency to the other—can be seen as something necessary to rhetorical success" (pp. 173–174). Understanding that self-disclosure requires making the body vulnerable calls for situating self-disclosure in an embodied, activist framework.

To do that, we draw from Vinson's (2017) notion of embodied exigence, a form of public activism in which individuals use embodied experiences of pregnancy to intervene in dominant narratives around teenage motherhood. For example, a pregnant teenager who receives condemning stares might enact embodied exigency by staring back, making a joke, or even calling out an unwanted physical or rhetorical act. This, we see, as embodied exigence evoking Royster and Kirsch's (2012) call to "tack in" to embodied experiences in order to "tack out" as a response to anti-feminist remarks and behaviors.

Rhetorics of self-disclosure build on Vinson's (2017) notion of embodied exigence by recognizing that infertility is an embodied experience that is complex, non-linear, and occupied by the body itself (as our own complex narratives throughout this chapter reveal). However, unlike embodied exigence, rhetorics of self-disclosure call for negotiations that make invisible bodies visible. While pregnant bodies (especially those that are non-normative or marginalized) are highly visible in public spaces and, therefore, create exigencies that enable feminist rhetorical interventions like those just described, infertility often goes unseen. Rhetorics of self-disclosure, therefore, call for interventions that uncloset infertility and that challenge social pressures to remain silent.

Further, self-disclosing one's experience with infertility and calling attention to that embodied, invisible exigency is not enough to support an activist agenda. Rhetorics of self-disclosure, we argue, are activist in that they make rhetorical space for others to self-disclose. In this way, there is no one dominant narrative of infertility. Therefore, self-disclosure invites others who have different narratives of infertility to disclose their experience and create an assemblage of experiences, aligning with Novotny's (2019) concept of counterstory.

Novotny (2019) draws on three infertility narratives that focus on what she calls non-normative infertility stories. These stories represent the lives of a trans teen encountering infertility for the first time, a gay couple identifying as infertile and seeking to build their family through surrogacy, and Novotny's experience with her own partner as they decide to decline fertility treatment and live child-free. These infertility stories act akin to an "antenarrative" (Boje, 2008) that opens up spaces for reinterpretation of dominant narratives. Drawing on the possibility of opening new spaces for the types of infertility narratives that are told, Novotny argues, then, for the queering of counterstories as a way to gather and acknowledge more nuanced, complex stories of infertility. Queering counterstory allows for an assemblage of multiple narratives; while these may contradict one another, they allow for a richer resistance of normative narratives—enacting moments for antenarratives to emerge.

One way we have seen such counterstories emerge is through Maria's work with ART of Infertility, a national arts organization that hosts workshops and educational and outreach events that portray the realities, pains, and joys of living with infertility. The mixed-media artwork and description shared below is just one example of how ART of Infertility participants use self-disclosure to create counterstories and embody exigencies that enable feminist rhetorical interventions. For example, the patient-artist who created the following piece, "Letting Go," used materials from her life prior to infertility and the shifts in identity that she had to reconcile after her diagnosis. The ceramic is a plate given to her as a wedding gift featuring her and her husband's initials in the center. As the artist's description reveals, she broke this plate to represent a fragmentation from the life she thought she and her husband would have with a child. The small glass pieces on the left side of the image are reused vials from past, failed fertility treatments. White gauze weaves around the ceramic attempting, yet with little success, to hold together the "traditional life" the artist thought she would have.

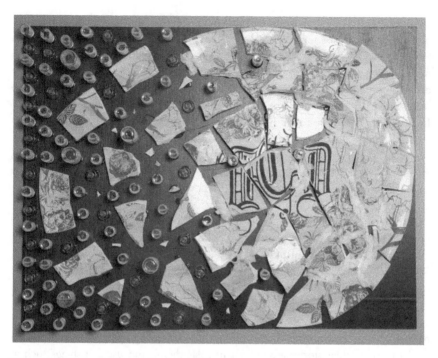

FIGURE 5.2 Denise Callen's "Letting Go"

Artist's description: "From childhood, we are brought up to believe in a traditional fairytale of how our lives will unfold: meet the handsome prince who steals the fair maiden's heart, marry and have a beautiful family. It can be a rude awakening when life veers from that path. Every plan I made revolved around this traditional view of how life was to play out. I married a wonderful man; we bought the perfect house with room for the traditional 2.5 children, and then the dream took us down a very dark path we never anticipated. Years of trying, expensive treatments over and over and over and over and over again, took their toll. Just when we would get good news, our hopes would be dashed with miscarriages and no heartbeats. I reached a point when it was time to stop crying, injecting, treating, and pouring money into a dream that wasn't to be. I needed to let go of the fantasy and find a new dream. I am now putting the pieces of my life together. Like this work, it is beautiful and holds parts of the past, but it is very different from the original plan. No matter how hard I try to patch it together, it, and I, will never be the same. I am stronger. I am wiser. I am happy. I am sad. I am living child-free."

Denise Callen

Denise's artwork is a form of self-disclosure that illustrates the embodied, non-linear nature of infertility. Her statement, for instance, that "I reached a point when it was time to stop crying, injecting, treating, and pouring money into a dream that wasn't to be. I needed to let go of the fantasy and find a new dream" represents the complexities of disclosing her infertility journey; she realizes that she will "never be the same" and will ultimately live "child-free." In this way, Denise's artistic rendering of her infertility journey offers a counterstory that challenges dominant narratives propagating the idea that infertility can (and perhaps should) be "resolved" through treatment. Self-disclosures like Denise's reveal how tacking in to one's embodied exigence and pushing back against normative ideals opens up new spaces for others to engage in infertility activism.

Another space where we see rhetorics of self-disclosure undergirding the kinds of embodied transformations and counterstories we discuss here is through infertility advocacy organizations such as RESOLVE. Every year in April, RESOLVE works with infertility partners to host a National Infertility Awareness Week, also known as #NIAW. The objective is to "change how others view infertility" and use personal stories as a method "to remove the stigmas and barriers that stand in the way of building families" (RESOLVE, 2018). Many patient-advocates participate in this campaign each year by blogging or using social media to share their stories around a particular theme and using hashtags such as #flipthescript, #listenup, and #startasking to signify their story as part of a national conversation. In 2018, RESOLVE partnered with Ferring Pharmaceuticals (a leading fertility pharmaceutical company) to encourage infertility advocates to share their stories by using the hashtag #TalkAboutTrying.

This is an effort to encourage individuals to draw from their embodied experiences of infertility, offer alternative narratives of fertility, and encourage others to share their stories and experiences. Initiatives like RESOLVE demonstrate how rhetorics of self-disclosure serve as an embodied, feminist rhetorical practice that makes visible the invisibility of infertile bodies. Our use of the word "rhetorics" in naming these practices as a form of feminist health activism is not accidental—indeed, we pluralize "rhetorics" when describing such self-disclosures in order to represent a multiplicity of lived experiences and to illustrate that infertility activism begins by making space for individuals to become aware of others' experiences. In this way, activism is not necessarily a political action, but a sociocultural and rhetorical intervention.

Infertility advocacy initiatives like #NIAW and #TalkAboutTrying illustrate how rhetorics of self-disclosure support cultural and rhetorical transformations that make infertility visible by encouraging individuals to share their stories and, in turn, to create space for others to share their counterstories and experiences. We see the need to make space for multiple stories of infertility. Making space for these multiple experiences, we argue, occurs through the sharing and self-disclosing of infertility, even when those stories do not reflect the same narrative.

Infertility Health Activism: Negotiating Shifting and Embodied Identities

When I first saw the CFP for this edited collection, I was thrilled. After almost four years of infertility, I had finally become comfortable with "outing" myself among colleagues and close friends (although I still struggled with self-disclosure with family members desperate for grandchildren); for me, this chapter and, indeed, this collection became an important space for rhetorically exploring my own emerging self-disclosures of infertility and how that informed my understanding of the broader infertility community and women's health activism. But then something happened. About halfway through our collaborative project, I became pregnant. I began to wonder: What does this mean in terms of my own infertility identity? Does becoming pregnant "erase" the emotional trauma of the past? Or change my contributions to this chapter? Or how I might remain an infertility activist?

Lori Beth

On a Saturday in March, I was in the car leaving a dentist appointment with my husband. Scrolling through my email, I saw a message from Lori Beth. It said:

"Hi Maria, I know you don't check facebook often, so I wanted to let you know that I've messaged you there. I sent it via facebook (rather than email) because it's personal in nature. LB"

Reading that message, an embodied response took over. I felt my blood pressure rise, my gut sink, and anxiety run through my nerves. I've felt this before, and while I did not know what Lori Beth needed to share, I became panicky. I quickly opened Facebook Messenger on my phone and read through the message. Lori Beth was pregnant. This was a surprise to her and to me, especially as we had spent the past few months talking and writing about our infertility experiences.

I took the day to process Lori Beth's news and in doing so, a new wave of anxiety rushed upon me—what about our writing? For months we had talked about the need to self-disclose our infertility, but now, how would she negotiate her infertility identity? How could we stay true to the premise of this chapter? Moreover, thinking about Lori Beth's pregnancy made me realize that I needed to negotiate my own infertility identity.

During the months of writing this chapter, my partner and I had made the decision to begin the domestic adoption process. We had told family and close friends—but I didn't tell Lori Beth. The adoption felt—and still feels—too uncertain. We have not been "matched" nor had our home study yet. So, in many ways, I still feel very attached to infertility as my identity. Yet, as we move further along in the adoption process, how will this change? Will I still identify as infertile? Such questions point to a key factor in infertility activism: it is embodied. And, so, it is in flux, always evolving and being negotiated through interactions with others.

Maria

As our above narratives reveal, self-disclosing infertility is not a singular narrative nor is the experience of infertility itself linear. Rhetorics of self-disclosure shift and change because they are not always anchored in a cohesive identity. In writing this chapter, for example, we chose not to erase our own embodied experiences of infertility by disclosing our evolving fertility and family statuses in the beginning of this piece; instead, we have made an explicit and intentional rhetorical move to let the organization of this chapter reflect and embody our own infertility identities as they unfurl. We argue that understanding how infertility shifts as an identity is key to understanding how self-disclosure acts as an evolving, embodied form of feminist health activism.

Johnson and Quinlan (2017) describe the complications around infertility identities, arguing that while an infertile individual may identify as an "insider" and a fertile individual as an "outsider," the boundaries around these identities are fluid and "fragile" (p. 4). In Lori Beth's case, her identity as an insider who experienced reproductive loss shifted once she unexpectedly became pregnant. And yet, this shift did not erase her infertility trauma or her desire to engage in infertility activism. In Maria's case, infertility is something she anticipates will be even more apparent because of her decision to adopt. Her body will not suddenly change and be read as a pregnant body. Rather, an infant will suddenly join her family and her future child will have a different birth story than most. Infertility, Maria anticipates, will always be somewhat publicly disclosed because of her family makeup. Rhetorics of self-disclosure, then, call for rhetorical strategies that allow for more dynamic and responsive forms of feminist health activism.

The ways in which individuals may identify and disclose their infertility status are also shaped by social and medical assumptions about how to treat or "cure" infertility. For example, after several years of not becoming pregnant, one of Lori Beth's family members suggested that she seek fertility treatment as a way to "resolve" her infertility. Lori Beth and her partner, however, had decided against this course of action. For many individuals, medical interventions into infertility (as well as the adoption of children) are an important means for achieving pregnancy or parenthood. However, these interventions also rhetorically position fertility and/or parenthood as a choice one simply need make. In other words, the perceived ability to *choose* parenthood makes invisible or, as Frost (2016) puts it, renders "unapparent" pro-natalist and misogynistic assumptions about women's ability to reproductively control their bodies. For many individuals, "fixing" infertility through treatments such as in vitro fertilization or through adoption is not an option, given the enormous costs and lack of workplace support (Farley Ordovensky Staniec, & Webb, 2007; Rycus et al., 2006; Smith et al., 2011).

Rhetorics of self-disclosure, then, make apparent the pro-natalist systems that regulate access to fertility care and support. Furthermore, the stories that we share above offer a more nuanced view of the complicated narratives that live within infertility activism. Infertility activism, as our stories demonstrate, requires a cultural shift in how reproductive loss is recognized, how "family" is defined, and how support is provided to individuals who find themselves reflecting on newly realized identities. To understand infertility activism through self-disclosure is to understand it as an action that interacts and lives within bodies and represents complex and shifting identities. Moreover, self-disclosure allows us to make visible these often-unexamined scenes of identity formation important to understanding how health activism operates.

Rhetorics of Self-Disclosure: Limitations and Affordances

Thus far, we have drawn from our own experiences, as well as from efforts by organizations like RESOLVE, to argue that rhetorics of self-disclosure provide productive spaces for engaging in infertility activism. However, we acknowledge that this framework can be a limited form of feminist health activism because self-disclosures in and of themselves might not necessarily yield specific healthcare policy changes or large-scale cultural shifts. While we believe this framework makes infertile bodies visible in public spaces and offers a counter narrative to public celebrations of pregnancy, we are cautious as to the extent of change it can produce.

For example, RESOLVE hosts an Advocacy Day that invites self-identified infertility advocates to travel to Washington, DC, to meet their local legislators and ask them to co-sponsor "fertility-friendly" bills. In meeting with these legislators, advocates are trained to share and self-disclose their personal stories with infertility and the challenges of building their families. While Advocacy Day has occurred annually for over ten years, legislative support for "fertility-friendly" bills has taken time, and congressional support remains static for introducing a bill that would mandate comprehensive fertility treatment coverage from insurance companies.

Despite the slowness with which political progress through organizations like RESOLVE has occurred, there have been some small, but notable legislative successes. For instance, in 2016, Veterans Affairs announced that VA-covered fertility treatment would be provided to Veterans with service-related conditions that resulted in infertility. The campaign to include veterans in the fight for reproductive justice was launched through the hashtag #IVF4Vets and received support through the Women Veterans and Families Health Services Act. Although the financial support for this act covers only fiscal years 2017 and 2018 (leaving the future security of this act uncertain), this legislative win for the infertility community demonstrates how public conversations about infertility can yield results that directly benefit infertile individuals and their families.

Another way in which rhetorics of self-disclosure might be limited is through social, cultural, and religious norms and ideologies that make self-disclosure riskier for some. Individuals who belong to certain religious, faith, or cultural communities may find it risky to divulge their infertility or reproductive loss either within or beyond the private sphere (Wiersema et al., 2006; Ali et al., 2011). Self-disclosure of infertility is also typically not as inherently risky as revealing other types of diagnoses such as HIV, cancer, or other serious illnesses. However, mental health studies (Gana & Jakubowska, 2016; Greil, Slauson-Blevins, & McQuillan, 2010; Jaffe, & Diamond, 2011) point to the extreme distress of an infertility diagnosis and the trauma of physically invasive fertility procedures. For instance, Steuber and High's (2015) study of the disclosure strategies of infertile individuals reports that "There are risks and benefits to disclosing private information, and it is important to note that revealing information, regardless of the strategy used, can result in negative outcomes." Self-disclosing infertility can, unintentionally, backfire and leave individuals vulnerable. It can result in the ending of or strain in relationships amongst friends, family, and partnerships, as well as identity challenges, a sense of loss of control, and feelings of isolation (Greil et al., 2010). The decision to self-disclose infertility in public scenes and spaces leaves one in a precarious position, opening them up for others to perceive them in a different light. Our call, then, for rhetorics of self-disclosure is tempered by our understanding that individuals must self-disclose infertility in their own ways, in their own time, and within the cultural contexts in which they live.

Like any other framework for health activism, rhetorics of self-disclosure operate within, and are limited by, the socio-cultural, institutional, and political systems of power that mediate them. Despite this reality, we see self-disclosure as a feminist rhetorical practice that directly intervenes in the silencing of infertility and provides a counterstory to celebratory narratives of pregnancy and childbirth. Such counterstories are needed because infertility as an experience of reproductive loss continues to go unnoticed. Yet we also recognize that some stories of infertility are heard louder and embraced more quickly than others. For example, stories that celebrate the "beating" of infertility and the need for women to cling to "hope" through numerous failed fertility treatments are often more visible than narratives of "failure," repeated reproductive loss, or the decision to live child-free. More work on what gets accepted as an "appropriate" self-disclosure about infertility needs to occur, whether it is comfortable or uncomfortable. Rhetorics of self-disclosure can help to begin that work.

References

Ali, S., SophieR., Imam, A.M., Khan, F.I., Ali, S.F., Shaikh, A., & Farid-ul-Hasnain, S. (2011). "Knowledge, perceptions and myths regarding infertility among selected adult population in Pakistan: A cross-sectional study." *BMC Public Health*, 11, 760–766.

Allison, J. (2011). "Conceiving silence: infertility as discursive contradiction in Ireland." *Medical Anthropology Quarterly*, 25(1), 1–21.

Arola, K.L. (2011). "Rhetoric, Christmas cards, and infertility: A season of silence." *Harlot: A Revealing Look at the Arts of Persuasion, No. 6*, Retrieved from http://mail.harlotofthea rts.org/index.php/harlot/article/view/83/73

Arola, K.L. (2014). "Pregnancy interfaced and inscribed." Paper presented at the Computers and Writing Conference (CWC)2014, Seattle, WA.

Boje, D.M. (2008). "Antenarrative." In R. Thorpe & R. Holt (Eds.). *The Sage Dictionary of Qualitative Management Research*, London: Sage, pp. 28–30.

Bute, J.J. (2013). "The discursive dynamics of disclosure and avoidance: Evidence from a study of infertility." *Western Journal of Communication*, 77(2), 164–185.

Ceballo, R., Graham, E.T., & Hart, J. (2015). "Silent and infertile." *Psychology of Women Quarterly*, 39(4), 497–511.

Centers for Disease Control and Prevention (2016). "Infertility." Retrieved from www. cdc.gov/nchs/fastats/infertility.htm

Cousineau, T.M., & Domar, A.D. (2007). "Psychological impact of infertility." *Best Practice & Research Clinical Obstetrics & Gynaecology*, 21(2), 293–308.

Farley Ordovensky Staniec, J., & Webb, N.J. (2007). "Utilization of infertility services: How much does money matter?" *Health Services Research*, 42(3p1), 971–989.

Frost, E.A. (2016). "Apparent feminism as a methodology for technical communication and rhetoric." *Journal of Business and Technical Communication*, 30(1), 3–28.

Frost, E., & Haas, A. (2017). "Seeing and knowing the womb: A technofeminist reframing of fetal ultrasound toward a decolonization of our bodies." *Computers and Composition*, 43, 88–105.

Gana, K., & Jakubowska, S. (2016). "Relationship between infertility-related stress and emotional distress and marital satisfaction." *Journal of Health Psychology*, 21(6), 1043–1054.

Greil, A.L., Slauson-Blevins, K., & McQuillan, J. (2010). "The experience of infertility: A review of recent literature." *Sociology of Health & Illness*, 32(1), 140–162.

Jaffe, J., & Diamond, M.O. (2011). *Reproductive trauma: Psychotherapy with infertility and pregnancy loss clients*. Washington DC: American Psychological Association.

Jensen, R. (2015). "From barren to sterile: The evolution of a mixed metaphor." *Rhetoric Society Quarterly*, 45(1), 25–46.

Johnson, B., & Quinlan, M.M. (2017). "Insiders and outsiders and insider(s) again in the (in)fertility world." *Health Communication*, 32(3), 381–385.

Johnson, M., Levy, D., Manthey, K., & Novotny, M. (2015). "Embodiment: Embodying Feminist Rhetorics." *Peitho*, 18, 39–44.

Novotny, M. (2019). "Infertility as counterstory: Assembling a queer counterstory methodology for non-normative bodies of health & sexuality." In W. Banks, M. Cox & C. Dadas (Eds.). *Re/Orienting Writing: Queer Methods, Queer Project*. Logan, UT: University Press of Colorado and Utah State University Press.

Pernot, L. (2015). *Epideictic rhetoric: Questioning the stakes of ancient praise*. Austin, TX: University of Texas Press.

RESOLVE: National Infertility Association. (2018a). RESOLVE Homepage. Retrieved from https://resolve.org

Royster, J.J., & Kirsch, G.E. (2012). *Feminist rhetorical practices: New horizons for rhetoric, composition, and literacy studies*. Carbondale, IL: Southern Illinois University Press.

Rycus, J.S., Freundlich, M., Hughes, R.C., Keefer, B., & Oakes, E.J. (2006). "Confronting barriers to adoption success." *Family Court Review*, 44(2), 210–230.

Smith, J.F., Eisenberg, M.L., Glidden, D., Millstein, S.G., Cedars, M., Walsh, T.J., Showstack, J., Pasch, L.A., Adler, N., & Katz, P.P. (2011). "Socioeconomic disparities in the use and success of fertility treatments: analysis of data from a prospective cohort in the United States." *Fertility and Sterility*, 96(1), 95–101.

Steuber, K.R., & High, A. (2015). "Disclosure strategies, social support, and quality of life in infertile women." *Human Reproduction*, 30(7), 1635–1642.

Ulrich, M., & Weatherall, A. (2000). "Motherhood and infertility: Viewing motherhood through the lens of Infertility." *Feminism & Psychology*, 10(3), 323–336.

Uthappa, N.R. (2017). "Moving closer: Speakers with mental disabilities, deep disclosure, and agency through vulnerability." *Rhetoric Review*, 36(2), 164–175.

Vinson, J. (2017). *Embodying the Problem: The Persuasive Power of the Teen Mother*. Brunswick, NJ: Rutgers University Press.

Wiersema, N.J., Drukker, A.J., Dung, M.B.T., Nhu, G.H., Nhu, N.T., & Lambalk, C.B. (2006). "Consequences of infertility in developing countries: Results of a questionnaire and interview survey in the South of Vietnam." *Journal of Translational Medicine*, 4, 1–8.

SECTION 2

Rhetorics of/and the Patient

The following chapters demonstrate the rhetorical, legal, corporate, and activist systems in which patients participate or struggle in terms of their health.

BRIDGING THE GAP IN CARE FOR WOMEN

Janeen Qadri

Women's anger about healthcare rights erupts in the media every few decades because, quite frankly, women, in my opinion, are sick of being treated like uneducated, naïve children. Women receive dismissive medical care, which is a very deep, systemic issue. In fact, many of my experiences lead me to believe that there is a serious mistrust between patient and doctor. Some of my medical experiences will shine a light on this perspective as a patient diagnosed with several health issues over the last four years. During this time, I've dealt with doctors who took me less than seriously—probably for many reasons that could include gender, educational status, or other reasons that are not evident to me. I offer three examples:

For over eight years before I was diagnosed with Celiac disease, doctors suggested that anxiety was the cause of my constant stomach pain, nausea, and extreme inflammation and bloating. I had never suggested nor was there any evidence that my mental state was suffering in any way. Yet, many doctors mistreated and downplayed my physical pain and the manifestations of what I felt.

Other poor experiences were at OBGYN offices. Some doctors did not take my constant pelvic pain seriously or thought I was promiscuous even though I have no history indicating that as a viable explanation. It turns out I have interstitial cystitis, which was diagnosed eight years after I first sought treatment.

Another frustrating appointment was with a doctor who refused to approve blood work that would aid in early detection of disease. I believe this was because the doctor prioritized the treatment of symptoms over seeking out their causes. I insisted on the blood work regardless, and the tests did come back positive for an autoimmune disorder. This knowledge has allowed me to be more proactive with supplements and lifestyle modifications, adjustments that could prevent triggering another autoimmune disease.

All of these negative experiences have actually led to my passion of being a patient advocate. Before dealing with symptoms of Lupus, I felt my purpose in life was to become a physician assistant (PA) focused on patient care. However, this diagnosis has changed the course of my future, and I couldn't be happier. Now, I can reach an audience directly because I am in their shoes. Having been in those shoes, I have learned a few things to share.

One way to improve patient/doctor relations that I've learned is to closely consider who I am speaking with so that I can communicate effectively. If the doctor is in a rush, I will state each symptom and ask for specific blood tests. If they make eye contact and ask more questions, then I know they will really hear my answer. And if a doctor cares enough to hear my answer, they will mostly likely think critically of appropriate testing. This is a 100% turn-around from the interactions of the past.

I have also shared my educational background with doctors: I have a bachelor's degree in health sciences. At times, this information leads to doctors who are intrigued to talk more openly with me about my health and my concerns.

Another solution I've found is to find ways to describe how symptoms affect me, so that they, as people without Lupus, but who might have had other pains and illnesses, can relate.

Finally, and most importantly, at the end of 2017, I co-founded Lupus Health Shop in hopes of reaching an audience of predominantly women who suffer extensively from Lupus and who have perhaps experienced the same type of poor care. It is not uncommon since Lupus is difficult to understand from a routine medical viewpoint.

Lupus Health Shop is an online database of free information on effective medical communication, legal working rights in the US, treatments that are safe while effective, and lifestyle changes that decrease severity and length of Lupus flare-ups and symptoms. Since some people with debilitating autoimmune diseases are stranded in their homes, online communication is most reliable.

To reach patients, I use social media such as Instagram to highlight how simple lifestyle choices and products can stop triggering symptoms. The ingredients in packaged food, skincare, haircare, and the pesticides on our produce are also direct triggers of symptoms. Environmental factors trigger disease, while genetics play a role in the probability of us carrying the trait of disease.

My goal is to bridge the gap between the patient and doctor. As I am in my infancy of reaching this audience, I hope to speak more on these matters at doctor-centered conventions as a patient advocate and offer free online educational classes and e-books on a variety of topics that include communication strategies, treatments, possible causes of symptoms, and healthcare as a whole to those impacted by autoimmune disease.

6

MAKING BODIES MATTER

Norms and Excesses in the Well-Woman Visit

Kelly Whitney

Each year, millions of women in the United States visit gynecologists, nurse practitioners, and family doctors for their annual check-up. Whereas women often refer to this check-up colloquially as their "annual" or "going for a Pap," in medical spaces, this check-up is commonly called the "well-woman visit." Typically, during this visit, women undergo a pelvic exam that screens for cervical cancer and a manual breast exam to check for lumps. Because of its focus on frequent, preventive screening, the well-woman visit has been credited with reducing cervical cancer mortality rates, establishing stronger doctor–patient relationships, and improving women's knowledge of their bodies and health. Indeed, the well-woman visit emerged in the 1950s primarily as an opportunity to screen women for cervical cancer, which was once the leading cause of cancer deaths in the US and has since dropped to fourteenth position on the list (NIH, 2013). Since then, the visit has also become a place for women to discuss other wellness concerns with their medical providers, including physiological health, sexual health, and family planning.

Despite the successes of the visit, health activists recognize that significant disparities exist between the visit's served and underserved populations. These disparities are evident in both who has access to the visit and who benefits from the visit's procedures. For instance, according to the CDC, cervical cancer affects women of color at significantly higher rates than white women, yet women of color are also, compared to white women, less likely to see a medical provider for an annual well-woman visit (US Cancer Statistics Working Group, 2018). The disparity between the medically served and underserved populations exhibits what Shildrick and Price (1998) call "the containment and excesses of the clinic." They explain that the clinic's practices and structures are based on "rigid categorisation of knowledge about being and the body" which "shape notions of what is proper and improper, normal and abnormal" about the patient's body (p. 10). What is presumed about the normal body is reflected in the clinic and its discourses, but unzipping such "corporeal closure" reveals the embodied excesses the clinic is unable to contain (p. 10).

In this chapter, I draw from Shildrick and Price's (1998) concepts of containment and excess to analyze biomedical discourses surrounding the well-woman visit and to trace whose bodies have come to matter in preventive gynecologic care. I use the terms *normal* and *excess* not to suggest bodies *are* normal or *are* excessive, but to highlight the normative work of biomedical logics that make bodies *emerge as* normal and excess. Those who exceed the norms affirmed by the practices of the visit can be identified by the well-woman visit's underserved populations, which materialize in terms of gender, age, race, sexual orientation, religion, body size, and socioeconomic status.[1] I argue that the boundary between the norm and excess is rooted in what Collins (1999) calls logics of eugenics: "The constellation of social policies, institutional arrangements, and ideological constructions that shape reproductive histories of different groups of women within different racial/ethnic groups, social class formations, and citizenship statuses" (p. 272). What was once an overt effort to eliminate certain populations through actual eugenics, such as forced sterilizations of women of color and women with disabilities, logics of eugenics continue to exist in cultural, political, and socioeconomic policies and procedures that are designed to serve some bodies and not, or even at the expense of, others.

While practices such as forced sterilizations are often recognized as eugenic methods, logics of eugenics are not always immediately recognized because they inform or structure policies and institutions and are, therefore, able to hide in plain sight. Thus, the well-woman visit, a common medical practice and "a fundamental part of medical care" that is "valuable in promoting prevention practices, recognizing risk factors for disease, identifying medical problems, and establishing the clinician-patient relationship" (ACOG, 2012) risks circulating eugenic logics because it continues to produce and underserve some women as "excess." Making apparent the eugenics logics that structure the well-woman visit is necessary for health advocates to promote inclusive, ingenious platforms that move toward an ethic of embodied difference.

The Well-Woman Visit: An Overview

While the specific components of the well-woman visit depend on each woman's needs and the medical providers' practices, a few objectives unify all well-woman visits. According to the US DHHS (2017), the visit has three objectives: first, to review the patient's health history, including her family's health and her sexual practices and health habits—information typically collected through an interview with the patient; second, to set health and wellness goals, which includes discussing and making plans regarding birth control and healthy living; third, to conduct a physical exam, which consists of a pelvic exam, a breast exam, and a Papanicolaou smear (often called a Pap smear or Pap test),[2] during which the provider uses a speculum to open the patient's vagina in order to see the cervix and collect cells to be tested for cancerous or precancerous cells.

Data on the number of well-woman visits each year is not available, but one way to track the frequency of preventive gynecologic care is through the number of pelvic exams performed annually. According to the CDC, 63.4 million pelvic exams were performed in the US in 2008 (as cited in Stormo, Hawkins, Cooper, & Saraiya, 2011). Though this data offers an incomplete picture of the frequency of the visit, it shows that it is a common, recognized medical practice that tens of millions of women in the US experience each year. Therefore, the well-woman visit is an important site for analysis of the complex relationships between language, power, and bodies, revealing "insights into ideological perspectives of the other that are extremely important in a healthcare industry that maintains persistent hierarchies and classes" (Melonçon, & Frost, 2015, p. 11) and intervening "into many of the problems plaguing our healthcare system" (p. 9). This chapter will make apparent the normative biomedical ideologies that circulate logics of eugenics in women's preventive health contexts as revealing such disparities is part of the work of rhetorical ingenuity in women's healthcare advocacy.

Biopower and Circulating Normalcy

To analyze the normative work of the well-woman visit, I draw on Foucault's (1978) concept of biopower and its role in normalizing bodies. According to Foucault, power structures codify knowledge *about* bodies and mark them as identifiable, recognizable, and categorizable subjects. While biopower is often associated as a function of the government (see Britt, 2000; Lay, 2000), others argue that biopower refers to discourses that govern bodies more generally. Stormer (2015) makes the case that "*government* refers generally to 'administration' or 'management,' not exclusively to the state, and potentially involves all public or private institutions and normative practices" (p. 29). Biopower, then, is not performed by a singular political entity, but can be performed by people and institutions that "determin[e] higher principles of how to live, which are presumably embedded within the order of everyday things and beings, and then putting those principles to work managing the conduct of people" (p. 30). Biopower doesn't work in a "top-down direction" on the public but "by enlisting them, often through communication, to participate in their self-management" (Scott, 2014, p. 110). Therefore, structures that govern how people live aren't limited to the state; medical discourses also participate in biopower by structuring how people live and what people value.

Medical structures play an important role in normalization processes because what is known about bodies becomes framed in terms of normal and "non-normal." For instance, body-mass indices published by influential organizations such as the NIH and the WHO categorize what counts as normal weight, underweight, and overweight. These categories, then, inform cultural perceptions of health and wellness that mark bodies as healthy and/or unhealthy. By enacting mechanisms of power and knowledge, medical practices and ideologies institutionalize biomedical notions of normalcy (Malacrida, 2009; Reaume, 2009). As scholars in critical race theory (Macey, 2009; Moreton-Robinson, 2006), disability studies (Dolmage, 2011; Michalko, & Titchkosky, 2009), and queer theory (Huffer, 2010; Slagle, 1995) have recognized, mechanisms of power and knowledge construct what counts as normal and non-normal bodies but also "sanctio[n] intervention into both in order to ensure conformity or bring into conformity, to keep or make normal, and also to effectively eliminate the threat posed by resisting individuals and populations" (Taylor, 2009, p. 53). In other words, becoming non-normal may conscript bodies for additional surveillance and control techniques such as frequent screenings, drug tests, welfare visits, and eugenics practices (Bridges, 2011; Enoch, 2005; Gurr, 2015). Such techniques are intended to "correct" non-normal bodies or ensure they are not a threat to those who are deemed normal.

Bearing in mind these relationships between biopower, bodies, and normalization, below I analyze medical literature on the well-woman visit spanning from the 1950s, when the well-woman visit began to emerge, through 2017, to: 1) identify patterns of what constitutes normalcy, 2) provide a comprehensive view of the ways the well-woman visit and women's bodies have been represented in medical discourse, and 3) trace the assumptions about them that circulate in biomedical discourse.

Becoming Excess Through Naming and (Dis)Identifying

The name "well-woman visit" creates excessive bodies because it carries biomedical understandings of both "well" and "woman." These terms hail some bodies to participate in the visit—which, in effect, normalizes these bodies—and makes excess those who disidentify with biomedical meanings of "well" and "woman." My goal here is not to criticize the name "well-woman visit," but to examine the normative work the name performs. Through the very nature of language as reflecting and deflecting, naming will always necessarily carve out boundaries, and this analysis examines how the particular terms "well" and "woman" come to signify, normalize, and make excess.

The term "well," as represented in medical literature, signifies in complicated ways. Through biomedical logics, the term "well" comes to mean "presumably" well. For example, a 1952 report on a study of the value of a well-woman clinic offers "asymptomatic well women of our community an opportunity to undergo a routine medical check up" (Latour, Oxorn, & Philpott, p. 439). It continues, "Only women who claimed to be free of complaints were admitted," which demonstrates selection criteria that reflects the types of bodies for whom the well-woman visit is designed: women who *identified as* and *felt* well (p. 439). The clinic reports that after four years, "Out of the total of 4,486 patients, 1,394 or 31% showed entirely negative findings. The remaining 3,092 women were discovered to have a total of 5,074 abnormalities" (p. 440). As this study suggests, just because women *feel* well doesn't necessarily mean they *are* well, according to biomedical understandings of "well." This distinction led one gynecologist to conclude, "The apparently well woman is not as well as we have supposed" and can be, instead, only "presumably" well (Siddall, 1956, p. 111).

The biomedical signifier "well" normalizes women who *identify as* and *feel* well but who also recognize that they are always only *presumably* well. Therefore, women who don't identify as or feel well (that is, women who may feel symptomatic) would see a doctor to treat symptoms, rather than seek out preventive screening. On the other hand, women who identify as and feel well but who don't see themselves as only *presumably* well may not feel the need for a preventive medical screening (because they already feel well). In this way, those who may not identify through biomedical meanings of "well" (that is, presumably well) become the excess of the "well-woman visit."[3]

The term "woman" in the title also creates excess by marking boundaries of who counts as a woman in this context. Specifically, "woman" signifies in the biomedical and reproductive sense since the well-woman visit originated in gynecology, a field focused on women's reproductive health, and more specifically in gynecology offices to screen women for cervical cancer. Since 1980, it has been known that cervical cancer is caused by HPV, a sexually transmitted infection. Because of its focus on reproduction, the well-woman visit has often been seen as necessary for women who are or are planning to become (hetero)sexually active. The well-woman visit, then, hails those who identify in these biomedical, reproductive ways and makes excess those who don't. Consequently, lesbian women (Brown, & Tracy, 2008) and transgender women (Dutton, Koenig, & Fennie, 2008) are included in the well-woman visit's underserved populations. These underserved populations reveal the rhetorical work of naming and belonging, and more specifically, what counts as "woman" in the well-woman visit.

Becoming Excess Through Practices and Knowledges

The boundaries between those who are invited to participate in the well-woman visit and those who aren't become further exacerbated when issues of access are taken into account. More specifically, in the well-woman visit, bodies that *make* medical knowledge diverge from bodies that *benefit* from medical knowledge. In fact, researchers regularly studied and experimented on bodies of color in order to learn more about human anatomy and to develop technologies and procedures that are commonly used in the visit. One of the most widely known instances of this phenomenon is J. Marion Sims, who invented the speculum and tested it by performing surgical experimentations on slave women. Washington (2006) claims that some physicians, including Sims, "bought and raised slaves for the express purpose of using them for experimentation" (p. 55). To develop his surgical procedures, Sims operated on the same women multiple times and, instead of administering anesthesia, relied on "the women to take turns restraining one another" (Washington, 2006, p. 65). To this day, the speculum remains a common device in pelvic exams.

Yet when the speculum design and surgical procedures were "perfected," it was white women who benefitted. According to accounts of the history of Mount Sinai St. Luke's Hospital, "Before coming to New York, J. Marion Sims developed the surgical procedure in the antebellum South. His first fistula patients were several African-American women who were slaves. These women—Anarcha, Betsy, Lucy, and others—made the new procedure possible" (Mount Sinai, 2017). As news of Sims' innovations spread, he "had established a world-wide reputation as a great surgeon and gynaecologist" as a result of "unethical experimentation with powerless Black women" (Ojanuga, 1993, p. 30).[4]

Sims (1866) claimed that his innovations were for the greater good of individuals, families, and the country. He wrote:

> From any point of view this subject is one of great importance; for the perpetuation of names and families, the descent of property, the happiness of individuals, and occasionally the welfare of the State, and even the permanence of dynasties and governments, may depend on it.
>
> *(p. 5)*

Yet his *means* of innovating reveal *who* and *what* matter and *when*. Washington (2006) succinctly explains this disparity: "Medical experimentation was profitable in terms of recovered health and life for whites, who benefited once the medical process had been perfected" (p. 54). In other words, black bodies mattered when they were used as research subjects that enabled medical scientists like Sims to develop technologies and practices, which, once perfected, failed to benefit black bodies to the same extent they would benefit white bodies.

A more well-known example of this racial discrepancy in when and how women's bodies have mattered in the well-woman visit's formation is the case of Henrietta Lacks. According to Skloot (2011), in 1951, Lacks, a black woman suffering from cervical cancer, had her cervical cells taken without her or her family's knowledge; these cells became the first that scientists could successfully reproduce in a laboratory without the cells dying. The cells, therefore, came to be seen as "immortal" and, because they could be reproduced rapidly, led to significant developments in cancer and AIDS research and enabled the development of vaccines (Caplan, 2013). Lacks died in 1951, yet her family learned two decades later that her cells lived on (Skloot, 2011). Moreover, because of the contributions her cells have made to scientific and pharmaceutical advancements, they "generated millions of dollars in profit for the medical researchers who patented [Lacks'] tissue" while her own family remained poor (NPR, 2010).

In these examples, black bodies matter to the extent that they provide knowledge to researchers for use in the development of technologies and procedures that benefit namely *not* bodies of color. According to the CDC, black women have the highest cervical cancer mortality rates at 3.3 per 100,000. For comparison, American Indian/Alaska Native women show a rate of 1.7 and white women a rate of 2.2. Hispanic women have the highest rate of cervical cancer at 9.4 per 100,000, compared to a rate of 6.0 for Asian women and 7.5 for white women (US Cancer Statistics Working Group, 2018). While low, these rates point to a larger pattern that despite the medical and technological advances made possible by the biological material of women of color, they continue to be disproportionately underserved by these same advances.

These racial discrepancies are part of medicine's wider troubled racial history. The twentieth century alone saw significant medical abuses that targeted bodies of color, including the US Public Health Service Syphilis Study at Tuskegee (CDC, 2015) and eugenics practices.[5] Because bodies of color have been targeted for abusive practices, many people of color became skeptical toward medicine (Washington, 2006). To participate in the well-woman visit, women willingly subject themselves to providers who hold power over them. This perspective toward biomedicine—a willingness to be screened regularly—accommodates bodies that have no reason to be skeptical of medicine. The bodies that do not submit to preventive screenings, perhaps because of historically abusive practices, aren't hailed by preventive medicine and therefore don't benefit from what biomedicine has to offer.

Becoming Excess Through Spaces and Places

The physical materials, spaces, and locations of the clinic also contribute to marking norms and excesses in preventive gynecologic care. Specifically, the bodies that are able to access and navigate the physical materials, spaces, and locations are those for whom the clinic is designed to serve. For example, climbing onto the gynecologic exam table, positioning their bodies in a way that cervical screenings are performed, or accessing the building by opening doors requires certain physical abilities. Similarly, the design and size of the exam table and medical gowns reflect normative assumptions about body size (Ahmed, Parr Lemkau, & Birt, 2002). Women who live in rural locations are also less likely to be screened because of access: The lack of health services and practitioners in rural areas lead women to have to drive long distances to seek screenings, which effectively lowers rates of attendance (Stewart, Thistlethwaite, & Buchanan, 2009). It's no surprise, then, that the well-woman visit's underserved populations materialize as women with disabilities (Mele, Archer, & Pusch, 2005; Nosek, 2006), overweight or obese women (Ahmed, Parr Lemkau, & Birt, 2002), elderly women (Blair, 1998; Calam et al., 1999), and women who live in rural locations (Stewart, Thistlethwaite, & Buchanan, 2009). Those who are unable to perform certain actions, navigate the space, or access the space, therefore, become excess since the clinic has not formed around these women's abilities or bodies.

Medical professionals often attempt to accommodate these excesses by developing innovative ways to offer preventive services. Two common strategies are: 1) to offer culturally tailored care through group visits for women of similar socio-economic status, and 2) for mobile clinics to travel to rural locations. While these approaches have the potential to make the well-woman visit more accessible, in practice, they often neglect important parts of the visit. One researcher explains: "The physical examinations are completed quickly. Each woman is offered a breast examination and a Pap test. Patients can ask personal questions, but a separate follow-up appointment is booked to discuss anything time-consuming" (MacKay, 2011, p. 126). In this example, women receive only one part of the well-woman visit. Education, counseling, and setting health goals, which are perhaps the practices that establish patients' longer-term relationships with health and wellness, are given less attention. Alternatively, some group visits and mobile clinics promote education and counseling but skip the pelvic exam, leaving women at risk for cervical cancer (Coughlin, & Rosenberg, 1983).

While attempts to make preventive care more accessible to underserved populations reflect medicine's commitment to serving all bodies, these efforts function as, to borrow a term from disability studies, *accommodations* because they attempt to retrofit a physical environment so others can participate (Michalko, & Titchkosky, 2009). This also extends to efforts to accommodate different body sizes and abilities, such as developing accessible exam tables, medical gowns, and speculums, all of which work towards making individual accommodations rather than designing an accommodating space (see Price, 2011). Similarly, retrofits reveal the assumptions about who uses the space. For instance, a wheelchair ramp makes buildings and other physical structures accessible to those in wheelchairs, but the need for the ramp itself reveals the designer's guiding assumptions and ideologies about the bodies that use that space, namely ambulatory people. The wheelchair ramp is an accommodation because it retrofits a space that would otherwise be inaccessible because the original design neglected to account for wheelchair users.

Toward an Ethic of Inclusive Activism

Advocates for women's preventive health practices and services have an ethical duty to recognize whose bodies are reflected and deflected in their platforms as well as the norms that these platforms circulate; such inquiries are rhetorically ingenious since they uncover that which would seem to be medically progressive as potentially problematic and damaging. Without this critical reflection, advocacy platforms risk codifying racist, classist, and ableist logics, as is the case with the well-woman visit. On the surface, advocating for the well-woman visit might appear moral and just because the visit is commonly accepted as helping women, but a closer analysis reveals the visit is rooted in narrow assumptions about whose bodies matter in preventive care. Ethical accountability in health activism—the practice of articulating the larger social and epistemological effects of one's activist platform, especially in contexts such as medicine that have been ascribed significant cultural and political power—must be a central concern of rhetorical ingenuity in order to work against, not perpetuate, logics of eugenics and embrace a medical ethic of inclusion. As such, stakeholders such as medical providers and researchers, patients, activists, and legislators have the capacity to *continue making* the well-woman visit what it is, which opens up possibilities for *what* preventive gynecologic medicine can be and *who* it can be for. By bringing attention to the normative work that medical practices and matters perform, stakeholders can recognize how they play a part in perpetuating norms and excesses. Therefore, I conclude this chapter with a call for inclusive activism that shifts assumptions from sameness to embodied difference.

The implementation of the ACA is one way that inclusive representation happens because it is founded on assumptions of embodied difference. This structural change to healthcare legislation recognizes that some bodies are disproportionately (dis)affected by traditional healthcare structures and responds to some of the root causes that have created barriers to accessing affordable, quality healthcare. Cost has prohibited many individuals from accessing healthcare, and so by expanding who qualifies for Medicaid, the ACA ensures medical coverage for those who are socioeconomically disadvantaged and, in so doing, removes a significant barrier that prevented some bodies from accessing care (which enabled these bodies to emerge as excess). Relatedly, the ACA prohibits systemic discrimination against traditionally vulnerable bodies. Specifically, women have traditionally paid more for healthcare services because of the types of services women require. Under ACA provisions, women can't be denied coverage, nor can they be charged more for healthcare that addresses women's specific needs (Lee, & Woods, 2013). The ACA has also addressed systemic discrimination by expanding coverage and improving access to healthcare to others who have become excess through systemic discrimination. For instance, the ACA recognizes that systemic discrimination against LGBT people made getting health coverage difficult and bans that discrimination (Stroumsa, 2014). Other studies have shown that more minorities have healthcare coverage, either through Medicaid expansion or private insurance, because of the ACA's individual mandate and ban on systemic discrimination (Chen et al., 2016).

While there are certainly limitations to and valid critiques of the ACA, the key point here is that the ACA assumes difference as in gender, socioeconomics, and sexuality and disrupts structural processes that neglect underserved populations by removing barriers to healthcare that existed because of narrow views of whose bodies mattered in access to healthcare. These structural changes allow more people, especially those who have previously been underserved, to participate in preventive healthcare. Consequently, the ACA makes important steps in rejecting logics of eugenics. Yet this movement toward a healthcare system committed to serving all bodies has been met with resistance. Political leaders have pursued efforts to repeal the law, claiming that the ACA prohibits consumer choice, invites government overreach, and creates financial burdens for individuals and businesses. While these are real concerns for many Americans and should be part of ongoing discussions and efforts in healthcare policy, there are also real, material consequences from decades of discrimination that must be at the center of any healthcare policy or reform. Privileging financial, small government, or consumerist commitments over coverage and access for all bodies risks returning to a system that invites only some bodies to participate in healthcare. By extension, any changes to healthcare policy that fail to guarantee comprehensive, affordable coverage to all individuals endorses eugenics logics. This is because only certain bodies that are afforded access to healthcare are served by a field that is tasked with keeping bodies healthy and alive.

As structural changes such as the ACA continue to change the composition of who accesses preventive care such as the well-woman visit, rhetorically ingenious activists can also embrace inclusive platforms and reject eugenics logics by presuming corporeal difference. This means that differences between women's material, lived experiences can inform advocates' cares, concerns, and arguments. One campaign that does this well is Care Women Deserve, a coalition of organizations committed to educating women on preventive care available to them through the ACA. Composed of representatives from the ACOG, the women's rights organizations United State of Women, UnidosUS, and Black Women's Health Imperative, as well as the National Women's Law Center, this coalition has developed a comprehensive, inclusive platform that presumes corporeal difference. Messages and infographics inform women of all races, ages, and sizes of services and procedures that they should consider; the group draws attention to its platform with the hashtags #CareWomenDeserve and #GetTheCare. Additionally, its website (http://carewomendeserve.org) offers a range of medical, legal, and cultural information and resources on women's preventive health, such as women's right to birth control under the ACA and guidance for appealing medical bills that should have been covered under the ACA. Between its social media hashtags and website, the campaign doesn't tokenize difference, but it does recognize that different bodies have different needs and provides information and resources that reflect these differences.

Such inclusive approaches to representation might even shift health advocacy goals. I echo Moeller and Jung's (2014) call for a shift in "responsibility for accommodating change … away from the individual and toward institutions and systems that currently enjoy the unchecked privileges of normalcy." This move requires efforts from institutions to the individual medical provider. To make the well-woman visit a viable preventative care measure for women, medical institutions—and medical regulatory and legislative entities—must recognize the normative work and, in turn, eugenics logics that medical practices perform and their effects on health disparities. Platforms centered on embodied difference might advocate for research and developments that serve all bodies.

Notes

1 I am not suggesting that bodies can, or should, be reduced to such classifications or categories. Because these categories are often used in the medical literature I surveyed, I use them throughout the chapter, attempting to trace how these subjectivities emerge and how they become excess through representations of practices and matters in medical literature. For closer analyses on how bodies become raced in medical settings, see Bridges (2011); Happe (2013).

2 Recently, medical organizations have endorsed Pap tests every 3–5 years rather than annually.

3 Recognizing the problematic term, one team of medical providers, when describing their clinic, state, "The title 'well woman clinic' was avoided so that women who regarded themselves as 'not well' may feel that they are welcome at the clinic" (Saine, Coupe, & Johnson, 1986, p. 86). This is the only instance in the medical literature I came across that addressed the implications of the title "well-woman" visit.

4 While many modern medical ethicists and practitioners have criticized Sims' methods, some defend his practices, claiming that his work was a product of his time (a southerner living in a time of slavery) and that his enslaved patients were "willing participants in his surgical attempts" to alleviate their "enormous suffering" (Wall, 2006, p. 346).

5 In the 1960s and 1970s, loosening sterilization regulations led to forced and coerced sterilizations of women of color. Enoch (2005) claims the "adjusted standards … enabled willing members of the medical community to adopt a Malthusian ideology that targeted minority groups and the poor as primary subjects for sterilization" (9).

References

Ahmed, S.M., Parr Lemkau, J., & Birt, S.L. (2002). "Toward sensitive treatment of obese patients." *Family Practice Management*, 9(1), 25–28.

American College of Obstetricians and Gynecologists (ACOG), The. (2012). "Well-woman visit. Committee Opinion No. 534." *Obstetrics & Gynecology*, 120(2), 421–424.

Blair, K.A. (1998). "Cancer screening of older women: A primary care issue." *Cancer Practice*, 6(4), 217–222.

Bridges, K.M. (2011). *Reproducing race: An ethnography of pregnancy as a site of racialization.* Berkeley, CA: University of California Press.

Britt, E.C. (2000). "Medical insurance as bio-power: Law and the normalization of (in)fertility." In M.M. Lay, L.J. Gurak, C. Gravon, & C. Myntti (Eds.). *Body talk: Rhetoric, technology, reproduction* (pp. 207–225). Madison, WI: University of Wisconsin Press.

Brown, J.P., & Tracy, J.K. (2008). "Lesbians and cancer: An overlooked health disparity." *Cancer Causes & Control*, 19, 1009–1020.

Calam, B., Norgrove, L., Brown, D., & Wilson, M.A. (1999). "Pap screening clinics with native women in Skidegate, Haida Gwaii." *Canadian Family Physician*, 45, 355–360.

Caplan, A. (2013). "NIH finally makes good with Henrietta Lacks' family—and it's about time, ethicist says." Retrieved from www.nbcnews.com/health/nih-finally-makes-good-henrietta-lacks-family-its-about-time-6C10867941

Chen, J., Vargas-Bustamante, A., Mortensen, K., & Ortega, A.N. (2016). "Racial and ethnic disparities in health care access and utilization under the affordable care act." *Medical Care*, 54(2), 140–166.

Collins, P.H. (1999). "Will the 'real' mother please stand up?: The logic of eugenics and American national family planning." In A.E. Clark, & V.L. Olesen (Eds.). *Revisioning women, health, and healing: Feminist, cultural, and technoscience perspectives.* (pp. 266–282). New York: Routledge.

Coughlin, M., & Rosenberg, R. (1983). "Health education and beyond: A Soviet women's group experience." *Journal of Jewish Communal Service*, 60(1), 65–69.

Dolmage, J. (2011). "Disabled upon arrival: The rhetorical construction of disability and race at Ellis Island." *Cultural Critique*, 77(1), 24–69.

Dutton, L., Koenig, K., & Fennie, K. (2008) "Gynecologic care of the female-to-male transgender man." *Journal of Midwifery & Women's Health*, 53(4), 331–337.

Enoch, J. (2005). "Survival stories: Feminist historiographic approaches to Chicana rhetorics of sterilization abuse." *Rhetoric Society Quarterly*, 35(3), 5–30.

Foucault, M. (1978). *Discipline and punish: The birth of the prison.* (A. Sheridan, trans.). New York: Pantheon.

Gurr, B. (2015). *Reproductive justice: The politics of health care for Native American women.* New Brunswick, NJ: Rutgers University Press.

Happe, K.E. (2013). *The material gene: Gender, race, and heredity after the human genome project.* New York: New York University Press.

Huffer, L. (2010). *Mad for Foucault: Rethinking the foundations of queer theory.* New York: Columbia University Press.

Latour, J.P.A., Oxorn, H., & Philpott, N.W. (1952). "An assessment of the value of a well woman clinic." *Canadian Medical Association Journal*, 67, 439–442.

Lay, M.M. (2000). *The rhetoric of midwifery: Gender, knowledge, and power.* New Brunswick, NJ: Rutgers University Press.

Lee, N.C., & Woods, C.M. (2013). "The Affordable Care Act: Addressing the unique health needs of women." *Journal of Women's Health*, 22(10), 803–806.

Macey, D. (2009). "Rethinking biopolitics, race and power in the wake of Foucault." *Theory, Culture & Society*, 26(6), 186–205.

MacKay, F.D. (2011). "Well woman's group medical appointment: For screening and preventive care." *Canadian Family Physician*, 57, 125–127.

Malacrida, C. (2009) "Discipline and dehumanization in a total institution: Institutional survivors' descriptions of time-out rooms." In R. Michalko & T. Titchkosky (Eds.). *Rethinking normal: A disability studies reader* (pp. 181–196). Toronto, ON: Canadian Scholars Press.

Melançon, L., & Frost, E.A. (2015). "Charting an emerging field: The rhetorics of health and medicine and its importance in communication design." *Communication Design Quarterly*, 3(4), 7–14.

Mele, N., Archer, J., & Pusch, B.D. (2005). "Access to breast cancer screening services for women with disabilities." *Journal of Obstetric, Gynecologic, & Neonatal Nursing*, 34(4), 453–464.

Michalko, R., & Titchkosky, T. (Eds.). (2009). *Rethinking normalcy: A disability studies reader.* Toronto, ON: Canadian Scholars Press.

Moeller, M., & Jung, J. (2014). "Sites of normalcy: Understanding online education as prosthetic technology." *Disabilities Studies Quarterly*, 34(4), Retrieved from http://dsq-sds.org/article/view/4020/3796

Moreton-Robinson, A. (2006). "Towards a new research agenda? Foucault, whiteness and indigenous sovereignty." *Journal of Sociology*, 42(4), 383–395.

Mount Sinai St. Luke's Department of Obstetrics & Gynecology. (2017). "History of the department." Retrieved from https://www.mountsinai.org/locations/st-lukes/about/history

National Institutes of Health (NIH). (2013). "Cervical cancer." Retrieved from https://report.nih.gov/nihfactsheets/viewfactsheet.aspx?csid=76

National Public Radio (NPR). (2010) "'Henrietta Lacks': A donor's immortal legacy." Retrieved from www.npr.org/2010/02/02/123232331/henrietta-lacks-a-donors-immortal-legacy

Nosek, M.A. (2006). "The changing face of women with disabilities: Are we ready?" *Journal of Women's Health*, 15(9), 996–999.

Ojanuga, D. (1993). "The medical ethics of the 'father of gynaecology', Dr. J Marion Sims." *Journal of Medical Ethics*, 19(1), 28–31.

Price, M. (2011). *Mad at school: Rhetorics of mental disability and academic life.* Ann Arbor, MI: University of Michigan Press.

Reaume, G. (2009). "Patients at work: Insane asylum inmates' labour in Ontario, 1841–1900." In R. Michalko & T. Titchkosky (Eds.). *Rethinking normal: A disability studies reader* (pp. 158–180). Toronto, ON: Canadian Scholars Press.

Saine, P.J., Coupe, J., & Johnson, H. (1986, February). "Well woman care." *Journal of the Royal College of General Practitioners*, 36(283), 86.

Scott, J.B. (2014). "Biopower and biopolitics." In T. Thomspon (Ed.). *SAGE encyclopedia of health communication* (pp. 110–113). Thousand Oaks, CA: Sage.

Shildrick, M., & Price, J. (Eds.). (1998). *Vital signs: Feminist reconfigurations of the bio/logical body.* Edinburgh, UK: Edinburgh University Press.

Siddall, A.C. (1956). "A new frontier in the private practice of gynecology." *Obstetrics & Gynecology*, 8(1), 107–111.

Sims, J.M. (1866). *Clinical notes on uterine surgery.* New York: William Wood & Co.

Skloot, R. (2011). *The immortal life of Henrietta Lacks.* New York: Broadway Paperbacks.

Slagle, R.A. (1995). "In defense of queer nation: From identity politics to a politics of difference." *Western Journal of Communication*, 59(2), 85–102.

Stewart, R., Thistlethwaite, J., & Buchanan, J. (2009). "Can rural practice nurses, physician assistants and nurse practitioners fulfill patient expectations regarding the 'well woman checks'?" Proceedings from the 10th National Rural Health Conference, Cairns, Queensland, Australia, pp. 1–12.

Stormer, N. (2015). *Sign of pathology: US medical rhetoric on abortion, 1800s–1960s.* State College, PA: Pennsylvania State University Press.

Stormo, A.R., Hawkins, N.A., Cooper, C.P., & Saraiya, M. (2011). "The pelvic examination as a screening tool: Practices of US physicians." *Archives of Internal Medicine*, 171(22), 2053–2054.

Stroumsa, D. (2014). "The state of transgender health care: Policy, law, and medical frameworks." *American Journal of Public Health*, 104(3), 31–38.

Taylor, D. (2009). "Normativity and normalization." *Foucault Studies*, 7. Retrieved from https://rauli.cbs.dk/index.php/foucault-studies/article/view/2636

US Cancer Statistics Working Group. (2018) "US cancer statistics data visualizations tool based on November 2017 submission data (1999–2015)." Retrieved from https://gis.cdc.gov/Cancer/USCS/DataViz.html

US Centers for Disease Control and Prevention. (2015). "The Tuskegee timeline." Retrieved from www.cdc.gov/tuskegee/timeline.htm

US Department of Health and Human Services (2017). "Get your well-woman visit every year." Retrieved from https://healthfinder.gov/HealthTopics/Category/everyday-healthy-living/sexual-health/get-your-well-woman-visit-every-year

Wall, L.L. (2006). "The medical ethics of Dr L Marion Sims: A fresh look at the historical record." *Journal of Medical Ethics*, 32(6), 346–350.

Washington, H.A. (2006). *Medical apartheid: The dark history of medical experimentation on black Americans from colonial times to the present.* Norwell, MA: Anchor.

7

DOULA ADVOCACY
Strategies for Consent in Labor and Delivery

Sheri Rysdam

Introduction

I am a teacher of writing, a rhetorician, a feminist, a part-time doula, and, when I began drafting this chapter, I was pregnant for the first time. Before entering into this new subjectivity of "pregnant woman," I believed that my education, professional experiences, and background would help me to navigate bureaucratic systems with more ease than some of my pregnant peers. My philosophy as a feminist, I thought, would help empower me to advocate for my best interests within these systems. Though nothing can replace first-hand experience of actually giving birth, I reasoned that my training and experience as a doula was educative and thorough. I was already familiar with childbirth: the stages, the behaviors, the sounds, the smells, the options, the common interventions and their outcomes, and the most common symptoms of fetal distress. However, even with this strong background knowledge, I could not successfully advocate for myself to have the kind of birth I would have liked to have had: a low-intervention homebirth.

My ideal birth was not some strange approach (not that there's anything wrong with that). My heart's desire for childbirth was fairly simple: It was informed by my past experiences and should have been available to me, but it was not. My own experiences illustrate that in childbirth, like so much of the lived, physical, female experience, options are limited, sometimes violently, by sexist bureaucracies and their practitioner enforcers. In this chapter, I look at the unfortunate link between violence and childbirth to theorize how doulas might employ rhetorical strategies to increase consent[1] and to protect women from violence in the medical system. A central argument of this chapter is that excessive medical interventions can inhibit consent and that doulas can help women to resist such interventions. Those strategies are: birth plans and stories, dialogic communication and concordance, strategic contemplation and rhetorical listening.

Birth Violence and Consent

Historically, women have been consistently violated in the process of receiving medical care. According to Rich (1976), this violence stems from "patriarchal technology," which "turned against woman her own organic nature, the source of her awe and her original powers" (pp. 126–127). Rich continues, "In a sense, female evolution was mutilated, and we have no way now of imagining what its development hitherto might have been; we can only try, at last, to take it into female hands" (pp. 126–127). In the hands of well-trained doulas (traditionally female), the childbirth experience might be much less violent.

From my experience, I know that many doulas in my community have witnessed women being told not to push because the doctor was not yet present. Worse, there are many stories of doctors holding the baby in until a woman agrees to comply with the doctor's proposed interventions. Commonly, a woman is laboring on her side or on hands and knees, and the doctor will ask her to move to her back—a position known for increasing pain in labor and inhibiting the benefits of gravity. When the laboring woman, in the final stages and pushing with contractions, doesn't comply, the doctor holds his hand to the woman's vagina and holds the baby's head in until she agrees to move into a position that is easier for the doctor. Several doulas in my community refuse to work with providers who regularly employ these violent tactics, but these are exactly the circumstances in which a good doula's presence is especially necessary. In the blur of childbirth, some women do not recall the violence, whereas doulas stand as witnesses, and they can and do share their experiences.

Many women are so used to having their bodies manipulated without their consent that they fail to experience these violences *as* violences. Additionally, if a woman experiences birth trauma, such as an episiotomy without her consent, frequently the care provider only has to say that the baby's life was in danger to quell any arguments or concerns that the new mother might have. What may seem horrific to a doula or birth worker who knows better might seem normal to a woman who has never experienced or witnessed childbirth. Of course, birth is intimate and somewhat unpredictable; there exists a wide margin for a "normal" childbirth experience. This reality poses a challenge for medical establishments, which increasingly rely on tools such as algorithms and protocols for decision-making. No doubt these save many lives from human error, but they also mean that women in labor, during what is a deeply physical, intense, and varied experience, are subject to hospital procedures that may or may not serve their unique experience.

Often, hospital protocols take precedence over the wishes, desires, and even consent of the patient. Anthropologists like Davis-Floyd (2003) have argued that in a "technocratic mode of care ... the human body is a machine," and "[w]ithin the techno-medical model of birth, some medical intervention is considered necessary for every birth" (p. 185). Seigel (2014) puts it another way:

The role of the user of the technological system of prenatal care—that is, the pregnant woman—is to work at disciplining her body and practices in accordance with public pregnancy narratives and to submit to the authority, guidance, and surveillance of medical professionals.

(p. 13)

When rigid protocols and medical interventions are considered a necessary and routine part of the childbirth experience, the wishes of the patient are not prioritized.

Wertz (1977) noted the benefits of movement during childbirth and the difficulties women might experience in contemporary birth postures: "Pain seems to be greatly reducible when persons are free to move their bodies to find a more comfortable position. For the restrained, body pain can be excruciating. Yet the modern delivery table prevented women from adjusting their position" (p. 197). Likewise, certain routinely used medical interventions, such as IV drugs like epidurals for pain, put women at a "fall risk." Once they've been administered, women have to stay on the bed, further limiting their mobility and, thus, the ability to get more comfortable during childbirth.

Kitzinger (2015) argues against unnecessary medicalization of childbirth. Kitzinger found that "behavior in hospitals is not always as rational and scientific as it seems and that a lot of action is heavily ritualized" (p. 167). In order to avoid the negative practices in hospitals:

Women choose homebirth largely because they wanted to be protected from interventionist obstetrics, could have one-to-one midwife care from someone they knew, and thought that they could bond more smoothly with their babies in a setting where stress was reduced.

(p. 167)

In that regard, depending on the care provider, women might also be safer from unnecessary interventions into the natural process of childbirth in a home birth. An example of an unnecessary intervention is the "husband's stitch" (p. 71), a practice that is still used today wherein doctors stitch up episiotomies and tears beyond the cut or tear in order to make the vaginal opening smaller, theoretically improving sexual enjoyment for men, but increasing sexual pain according to many women—including Kitzinger, who had the "husband's stitch" against her wishes after her first birth.

The "husband's stitch" is a strong example of why advocacy and strategies for consent are needed—women need to be protected in the vulnerable space of labor and delivery—especially in a culture that understands the value of technologies and bureaucracies better than it understands that individuals have a say in what happens to their bodies. To address this injustice, birth doulas—often invited to be present at hospital births—are in particularly advantageous roles to function as mediators for consent within the medical industrial apparatus and to offer rhetorical strategies for maintaining consent during childbirth. Doulas can employ the following rhetorical tactics: encouraging the writing of birth plans and birth stories, dialogic communication and concordance, and strategic contemplation. These moves could help women by promoting consenting exchanges between patient and healthcare provider. Each will be explained in turn in the following section.

Birth Plans and Stories

One rhetorical means of facilitating consent during labor and delivery is through birth stories. Sharing narratives function to increase birth literacy which, in turn, empowers interlocutors. Lay (2000), for example, argues that women use "one another's birth stories to enhance their understandings of their craft, to debate proper procedures and interventions and, where possible, to find common ground with other practitioners" (p. 68). Hensley Owens (2015) writes about childbirth as a way to regain power in what feels like a very disempowering system. She begins by telling the story of her own birth, which almost occurred in a Volkswagen bus because the actors involved failed to take her mother seriously. She writes that her mother had to assert "her rhetorical agency twice before anyone ... fully believed or acted upon the message that she was in labor" (p. ix). Stories of this nature pervade narratives of the childbirth experience, illustrating just how little women are trusted to make decisions, to trust experience—even when it comes to the childbirth that is happening to their own bodies. Hensley Owens writes, "Women absorb, respond to, and share many kinds of childbirth stories, with a variety of rhetorical and material effects that extend far beyond childbirth itself" (2015, p. x), making birth plans a feminist rhetorical act. Yet, she notes that attempts to reclaim agency do not always work in childbirth, and she considers this a failure of feminism (p. 10). Not only are women routinely met with skepticism or distrust, the authority of the doctors and science consistently outweighs the authority of a woman in labor. Doulas are a promising space to think through how women might overcome seemingly insurmountable obstacles to being taken seriously as rhetorically authorized subjects in labor and delivery.

Hensley Owens argues that birth plans (many of which are now shared via online forums) are an attempt for women to regain power in childbirth. She claims they are an example of attempted feminist rhetorical agency—"attempted" because the outcomes are not always "positive" in that women are sometimes (often) still disempowered during childbirth: "The genre of the birth plan is relatively new and has fairly explicit rhetorical intentions: women write birth plans to claim agency, to some extent, over the circumstances of labor and delivery" (2015, p. 39). She later adds, "Birth plans, a written form of resistance, work together with women's voices to codify particular resistances" (p. 88). Birth plans help facilitate consent and agency. The emergence of the birth plan as a genre indicates a reclaiming of agency in the childbirth process—a process that has been too often removed from women's wisdom and experience and replaced with medical authority. If birth plans work not by giving women stronger agency, but by educating women on their options, doulas strengthen this outcome and make it more likely that women will take what they learn and insist on the kinds of birth experiences they wish to have.

Dialogic Communication and Concordance

Segal (2008) offers "concordance" as a way of navigating the healthcare system in general, and the strategy can especially be applied to medicalized childbirth. Segal reminds us,

> We have not ... really received *orders* from our doctors; we have received *advice*. We stand, then, needing to be persuaded. ... We may cooperate more readily when we participate in decision-making and when prescriptions accord with our health beliefs.
>
> *(p. 149)*

In this way, Segal uses a rhetorical strategy to help patients move from strict compliance to the system's rules, toward concordance, a two-way agreement on how to proceed.

This type of agreement is necessary because currently, too often, women are not consenting to these procedures. Wolf (2001) recalls an interview with a midwife who said,

> I have never yet seen a physician show the respect of informing a woman of what is required—"I need to do this procedure"; instead they just cut, often without even telling the woman—sometimes when the baby is just about born; sometimes the husband is shouting for the doctor to stop. Many women find this cut the most traumatic part of the birth. Yet episiotomy is seen in the same light as taking a temperature—it's that routine.
>
> *(p. 193)*

In fact, over time, my role as a doula has increasingly become one of advocacy; I help facilitate consent. Perhaps there is no other place where women's bodies are physically acted upon than in a typical hospital setting during childbirth. It is not uncommon for nurses to approach a woman, stating, "Let's get an IV in you." Proclamations are made: "We need to break the bag of waters," "We might need to section her," and "Up the pit" are all common phrases heard throughout the labor and delivery floor. These phrases or commands do not allow for dialogic communication or concordance, which involves a mutual decision about the care plan and procedure. In part, this happens because the process is oftentimes so very routine for these workers. But, it's also because the US medical apparatus often wields unchecked power resulting in the objectification of women's bodies.

Too often in medicalized childbirth, individuals lose sight of their own autonomy. It makes sense that one weighs their own personal desires, gauges their own personal bodily risks and benefits along with the suggestions of the practitioner, even as they are informed by the larger bureaucratic medical institution's policies. Doulas can facilitate concordance by clearly asking questions of both the care provider and the patient.

Strategic Contemplation and Rhetorical Listening

In addition, strategic contemplation is a rhetorical strategy that "allows scholars to observe and notice, to listen to and hear voices often neglected or silenced, and to notice more overtly their own responses to what they are seeing, reading, reflecting on, and encountering during their research processes" (Royster, & Kirsch, 2012, p. 85). A doula's role here can be in witnessing, supporting, sharing stories, and facilitating the meaning making of it all.

Similarly, Ratcliffe's (2005) "rhetorical listening" is a rhetorical *techne* that can be used to facilitate consent in medical situations, especially childbirth: "Rhetorical listening may be employed to hear people's intersecting identifications ... the purpose being to negotiate troubled identifications" (p. 18). Certainly, there are "troubled identifications" between the actors (patients, midwives, doctors, bureaucracies, etc.) involved in the medicalized childbirth setting. Ratcliffe's rhetorical listening functions to facilitate "productive communication" (p. 25). Rhetorical listening is a strategy that is often used for those seeking to improve communication. After all, those who are most disadvantaged by a communication are most likely to seek improved communication through rhetorical strategies, and those people tend to have less power in the rhetorical exchange. So, many of the rhetorical strategies that are available as means of effective communication are not used by those who need it most (medical doctors) or entities with the most power (medical institutions). Instead, the burden and risks involved with communication in medical settings lies more with the patient.

A kind of reciprocal communication is required for rhetorical listening. If one side of the conversation has less incentive to create effective communication, as is the case in medicalized childbirth, the communication will obviously be less effective. Those entities with more power (such as medical establishments) do, however, have some incentive for communication in order to establish a good reputation, avoid litigation, and improve birth outcomes, for example, and that incentive needs to be amplified in these rhetorical communications. As such, the effective use of dialogic communication (Kent, & Taylor, 2002), wherein every relevant channel is negotiated, can be an effective strategy for facilitating consent.

How Doulas Might Employ Rhetorical Strategies for Consent

Doulas can employ these rhetorical strategies in the childbirth setting. Birth doulas provide non-medical labor assistance to women during childbirth. Although doula work frequently entails comfort measures such as counter pressure, massage, and words of encouragement, increasingly, because consent is not well understood, the doula's role is also one of advocacy. Doulas can teach and enable conversations that cultivate an ethos of consent within the medical industrial complex and more broadly. In doing so, they can create a cultural shift in how women navigate healthcare systems.

In a more traditional doula relationship, doula and client have educational meetings and bond to some extent in advance of labor and delivery, and the doula typically meets with the woman at least one more time postpartum. In this traditional relationship, the doula can better manage the channels of a dialogic communication, which unfolds over time. The doula is well aware of the patient's background and can best help facilitate her birth plan during child-birth. Because consent is often not implicit or widely practiced, this doula work provides a critical avenue for understanding and facilitating an ethos of consent for these women during labor and delivery. In addition to traditional comfort measures, doulas now have an important role in making consent a key aspect of a feminist medical rhetorical practice.

When one sees women's bodies as people with agency and is concerned with consent, these phrases and mandates change their tone and purpose to become actual questions for the patient, which she is at liberty to answer truthfully. In a consenting exchange there are at least four parts: the provider gives information about the procedure, they give an explanation of why the procedure is recom-mended, space is provided for questions or concerns, and finally request for permission to proceed is made.

Like the earlier example of the doctor who gave the woman an episiotomy despite her pleas, I have witnessed similar violations where consent was not established. In fact, one must only attend a few labors before witnessing these grave violations. Imagine supporting an unmedicated, laboring mother, who had an episiotomy without her consent just before the baby was born. The laboring mother has requested no medicine and no episiotomy in her birth plan. In the intense final moments of childbirth, the midwife engages the husband in eye contact, lifts the scalpel, and raises her eyebrows as if to ask, "Is this ok?" The worried husband, clutching his partner's leg, nods approval, though he knows his wife wanted to tear if necessary, instead of sustaining a surgical cut. He thinks this must be the only option. Consent has not been sufficiently established. The perineum is severed, and the baby is born after a few more pushes.

As a doula, my job is also to help women process their birth, and their trauma if necessary, but not to introduce trauma. Afterward, using strategic contempla-tion, I can ask the woman how she felt about her delivery. She is usually obsessed now and smiling at her new baby; she is happy. So, although I might know, as a trained professional, that the midwife should have gained consent before administering the episiotomy, if the patient was not disturbed, I will not introduce trauma by bringing it up. Commonly, these types of traumas sink in over time, as strategic contemplation occurs, and women are able to process their birth. Often, they realize that things could have and should have been different.

Although doulas do not provide medical advice or administer any medical procedures, they can and do try to catch an unconsented procedure before it happens. When the midwife has the quiet exchange with the husband to indicate that she is about the cut the woman, a doula can advocate by saying, "It looks like you're considering an episiotomy," to the midwife. Then, the doula will turn to the patient and say, "It looks like they're considering an episiotomy. Would you like to discuss your options?" Sometimes the woman reaffirms that she does not want the episiotomy. Other times she agrees to the procedure, usually in no condition to "discuss." Frequently, and ideally, this intervention slows down the process. A conversation (although it may be brief) can happen and concordance can occur. An opportunity to establish consent emerges, and either way, the woman usually leaves her childbirth experience feeling more empowered and less traumatized than if she had been acted upon physically without her consent during her delivery.

Wolf (2001) argues that "The medical establishment too often produces a birth experience that is unnecessarily physically and psychologically harmful to the women involved" (p. 6). In her study, "A number of women who had given birth described a moment at which they felt the medical institution simply took over; oblivious to the mother's wishes, experience, or concerns" (p. 149). She continues, "I heard comparable ordinary traumas among many women I talked to—what I have come to call 'ordinary bad births'" (p. 145). Wolf's antidote to birth violence is midwifery care. She writes, "Midwives working on their own terms do not try to guide births along a path determined by unnecessary medical interventions. Rather, midwives wait, encourage, and prepare the way, successfully keeping medical intervention to a minimum" (p. 151). In fact, Wolf likes the birth center setting, where women have more time for nurturance, and dialogic communication is a key aspect of the exchange. Wolf is emphatic: "Women carrying babies must be nurtured and supported intensively" (p. 114). In the birth center, women often have access to both a more woman-centered delivery, but also more extensive medical intervention. However, Wolf warns against in-hospital midwives and birthing suites, which she argues serve as a kind of bait and switch and essentially have the same or similar outcomes as birthing in a typical hospital. The hospital's protocols are so rigid that very few women are actually able to labor within the institution's guidelines and end up delivering in Labor and Delivery, with a midwife who has to proceed very much like an OB and where the risk of cascading interventions is just as high.

In Wolf's own experience, she started in the birthing suite, but her birth eventually escalated to a cesarean section in an operating room. During her second pregnancy, her doctor said, "You had to be sectioned last time. You probably have an unusually narrow birth canal. Maybe your body just is not made to have babies." She continues, "my doctor wanted to be right about my being in need of his surgical help more than he wanted to heal" (p. 278). Thus, she illustrates once more the need for a strategy for consent and advocacy within a system that so typically distrusts and disempowers women's bodies.

Rhetorical Strategies in Action

I became pregnant after several years of volunteering as a doula and working on scholarship in feminism and the rhetoric of health and medicine. I offer parts of my birth story in this chapter to demonstrate how these rhetorical strategies can play out.

After a positive pregnancy test, I called my OBGYN, a woman with whom I have a good rapport and whom I have seen for several years. During that first phone call, the office staff told me they needed bloodwork to confirm my pregnancy. Once my pregnancy was confirmed, I had a first appointment where I was told I would have various screening tests. I would also be given an ultrasound to confirm the pregnancy and ensure it was not ectopic. None of this seemed necessary to me. I felt healthy and normal and pregnant. I also felt excited. I wanted to talk to someone about the strange new feelings in my body and my hopes and expectations for this journey. I thought my OBGYN would be the perfect person for this conversation.

At my early OBGYN appointments, despite my work in advocacy and consent, I already found myself compromising and feeling the need to "go with the flow" at the OBGYN's office, such as submitting to blood tests. I did not want to establish myself as a difficult patient. After all, maintaining a positive relationship with my doctor could improve the care I would receive during a time when so much was at stake.

At the appointment, I told nurses that I was opting out of the ultrasound. Even still, the OBGYN's routine was entrenched, and she assumed the normal practice of bringing the ultrasound machine into the room. Despite my declining of the ultrasound, the doctor continued into the room with the machine. She explained that she needed to confirm my pregnancy, my due date, and that the pregnancy was not ectopic. I told her I did not think those steps were necessary for me, and I wanted to skip them. Immediately, I felt at odds with the establishment. I was astonished by how hard I had to work to maintain a positive interaction while advocating for my wishes.

I also revealed my hope for childbirth: If all went well, I would labor and deliver my baby at home. However, having attended several births lasting more than a day, I was also well aware of some of the benefits of epidurals and other interventions in long labors. I wanted to have access to that care if needed. On one hand, if my labor lasted 8 to 10 hours, progressed steadily, and if I was managing the pain well (something I had frequently observed as a doula), why not stay in the comfort of my own home with a midwife, eating my foods, using my bathroom, and avoiding the cascade of interventions that can occur in a hospital?

Knowing that induction increases the rate of cesarean section and that first-time moms gestate on average for 41 weeks and 3 days, I asked how long I could be allowed to gestate in her care. She answered that after 41 weeks I would be monitored daily and possibly allowed to go as long as 42 weeks, though I got the distinct feeling this almost never happened. However, throughout the appointment, I was repetitively warned against the dangers of my pregnancy with comments such as "your placenta just gets too old and can't sustain life at that point." In this way, the OBGYN used our appointment time to warn against the dangers of pregnancy and childbirth, reaffirmed that she was uncomfortable with homebirth, and even shared a few horror stories. Generally, no person is more concerned with the health and welfare of their baby than the parents, and healthcare professionals need not spend so much time fear mongering pregnant women. For the most part, pregnant women are trying to make the best decision for themselves and their babies. The new flood of hormones that sustain pregnancy also tend to make women hypervigilant about safety and possible dangers. Warnings from healthcare professionals about everything that can go wrong can come across as emotionally manipulative. With this pressure, I could not establish the kind of dialogic communication that I hoped for.

It is true that many women enter childbirth with fears of hospitals or needles, or they worry that something bad will happen to their babies or worry about pain. After my experience as a doula, my biggest fear is of being violated by medical interventions with and/or without my consent. That is by far the most common trauma I have witnessed and the one I wanted to guard against if at all possible. Yes, things go wrong with the body, but in my experience, things go wrong through intervention far more frequently. Fears are not always rational, but research bears this out—many European countries have far better outcomes with fewer interventions.

Therefore, after my first interactions with the OBGYN, I decided to establish a relationship with a well-known, highly recommended homebirth midwife who had all the necessary certifications and decades of experience. The appointments were hour-long, rambling sessions, where I sat on a comfortable couch. Concordance was much more achievable in this setting. For example, I was given several different options for taking the glucose test, a routine test to check for gestational diabetes, which otherwise involves drinking a glucose solution to achieve a hypoglycemic episode, as is the standard practice of care in more traditional medical settings.

However, to be fair, these appointments with my midwife were not perfect. In fact, she also shared horror stories, but they were less related to my choices and more relayed as interesting anecdotes. I still did not want to hear them and sometimes had to remind her of that. However, it was much better than the chaotic, short visits at the OBGYN, where the predominant message was that the process of making a baby was dangerous.

During my fourth month of pregnancy, my OBGYN officially "fired" me. She said she was not comfortable with my desire for homebirth and was not willing to continue working with me if I chose to also see a midwife. My insurance paid 100% for the OBGYN and 0% for a midwife. My hope was to do some prenatal work through the OBGYN since the out of pocket costs for the midwife would have been prohibitively expensive. I could have proceeded with this plan unbeknownst to the OBGYN. She may have only noticed when I failed to show up for birth at the end. However, I was honest with her, and she refused to participate. My preference to have co-care throughout my pregnancy proved impossible, failing less than halfway through my pregnancy.

Accordingly, I now identify with Hensley Owens (2015), who writes about her own birth experience: "[T]he birth I wanted was most readily achievable at home ... I wanted options that a hospital birth simply could not provide" (p. 147). She gave birth at home and says her own birth choices were deeply informed by birth stories shared by other women, in addition to the "sanctioned experts" (p. 160). Like Hensley Owens, I found that the best birth option for me was not available, and homebirth would come closest to meeting my preferences. Still, like many other women, I did not have the resources or health insurance coverages necessary to make that goal an option. Left with a hospital birth and all of its attendant interventions, I needed a doula to help me to craft the birth experience I wanted to have. That said, if doulas like my own were trained in the rhetorical strategies I describe in this chapter, perhaps my own birth story would be an even more compelling example of agency in labor and delivery.

In my recent experience giving birth, with the help of my own doula, concordance was achieved with almost every decision, and my labor and childbirth experience was mostly a positive, loving, and exciting time. Still, I struggled with having to wait to push to accommodate hospital staff shift changes. Doulas as advocates for women's consent in birth, then, could be strengthened by strategic rhetorical work; this chapter is a move in that direction.

My own experience as a doula and new mother illustrate just how much agency and consent is lacking in the US childbirth experience, but it also shows how the use of rhetorical strategies can help to alleviate some of these issues. As Rich (1976) writes,

> As long as birth [...] remains an experience of passively handing over our minds and our bodies to male authority and technology, other kinds of social change can only minimally change our relationships to ourselves, to power, and to the world outside our bodies.
>
> (p. 185)

My hope is that promoting doulas as advocates can decrease negative incidences in childbirth. Because not every birthing person has access to the rhetorical strategies described in this chapter, doulas and other birth workers can use them to increase birth literacy, to help establish true consent, and to eliminate trauma and violence in the childbirth setting.

Note

1 Throughout this piece, the term "consent" refers to any situation in which a doctor or medical practitioner would be expected to ask permission and/or discuss the consequences, risks, and benefits of a procedure with the pregnant or laboring woman.

References

Davis-Floyd, R. (2003). *Birth as an American rite of passage.* Berkeley, CA: University of California Press.

Gaskin, I.M. (2003). *Ina May's guide to childbirth.* New York: Bantam Books.

Kent, M.L., & Taylor, M. (2002). "Toward a dialogic theory of public relations." *Public Relations Review*, 28(1), 21–37.

Kitzinger, S. (2015). *A passion for birth: My life: anthropology, family, and feminism.* London: Pinter & Martin.

Lay, M.M. (2000). *The Rhetoric of midwifery: gender, knowledge, and power.* New Jersey, NJ: Rutgers University Press.

Owens, K.H. (2015). *Writing childbirth: Women's rhetorical agency in labor and online.* Carbondale, IL: Southern Illinois University Press.

Ratcliffe, K. (2005). *Rhetorical listening: Identification, gender, whiteness.* Carbondale, IL: Southern Illinois University Press.

Rich, A. (1976). *Of woman born: Motherhood as experience and institution.* New York: Norton.

Royster, J.J., & Kirsch, G.E. (2012). *Feminist rhetorical practices: New horizons for rhetoric, composition, and literacy studies.* Carbondale, IL: Southern Illinois University Press.

Segal, J.Z. (2008) *Health and the rhetoric of medicine.* Carbondale, IL: Southern Illinois University Press.

Seigel, M. (2014). *The rhetoric of pregnancy.* Chicago, IL: University of Chicago Press.

Wertz, R. (1977). *Lying-In: A history of childbirth in America.* London: Macmillan.

Wolf, N. (2001). *Misconceptions: truth, lies, and the unexpected on the journey to motherhood.* New York: Doubleday.

8

GENDERED RESPONSIBILITY

A Critique of HPV Vaccine Advertisements, 2006–2016

Erin Fitzgerald

Introduction

There are approximately 14 million individuals newly identified with HPV—a sexually transmitted infection—in the US each year (Satterwhite et al., 2013). HPV causes cancer of the cervix, vulva, penis, anus, and oropharynx (Meites, Kempe, & Markowitz, 2016). Gardasil, developed by Merck pharmaceuticals and released on the global market in 2006, and Cervarix, developed by GSK, are two FDA-approved vaccines that provide protection against specific types of HPV linked with cervical cancer and genital warts (Meites, Kempe, & Markowitz, 2016). While both vaccines are marketed for women, only Gardasil developed a vaccine marketed for men, which was approved by the FDA in 2009 and became routinely recommended for men in 2011. Ad campaigns, though, overemphasize cervical cancer.

According to the Workowksi & Bolan (2015), 62.8% of women and/or girls and 49.8% of men and/or boys have received at least one of the HPV vaccines. However, HPV vaccine rates for young adults remain lower than other vaccines routinely recommended for teens in the US (Brown, Gabra, & Pellman, 2017). The most common reasons for getting an HPV vaccination are physician recommendations and the belief that the vaccine is mandatory; meanwhile, the main reasons for low HPV vaccination rates are the desire for more research on the vaccine, the vaccine's effect on sexual behavior, and low perceived risk of HPV infection or perceived lack of direct benefit from the vaccine (Holman et al., 2014; Brown, Gabra, & Pellman, 2017).

This chapter critiques Merck's marketing strategies aimed at increasing HPV vaccinations in young people with an emphasis on increasing its use in young women. Broadly speaking, health messages about vaccines are designed to increase audience awareness of disease prevention (Parrott & Condit, 1996), but such messages portray, in most cases, women as solely responsible for preventing disease via vaccinating themselves and their children. By framing HPV rhetorically as primarily a female issue, the discourses on HPV and its vaccinations become limited, depriving parents of the necessary information to make informed health decisions for their children regardless of gender.

Merck's Gardasil campaign over time, when read through the lens of "embodiment" (described below), reveals a reinforcement of assumptions about female responsibility, parental obligations, and heteronormative ideologies. In this chapter, I use three representative Gardasil campaigns from 2006 to 2016 to reveal these assumptions. The launch of the 2006 "One Less" campaign represents the first message that specifically targets female public audiences, establishing the narrative of HPV rhetoric on a national level. Implemented in 2011, "Third Time's a Charm"—a campaign considered successful by Alabama public health providers—provides a glimpse into HPV rhetoric at a local level. And, finally, the 2016 "Did You Know—Mom, Dad?" campaign captures the inclusion of both female and male public audiences at a national level for the HPV vaccine, which still reinforces a problematic narrative of female responsibility for private and public health. Ultimately, I argue that the rhetoric of HPV marketing situates the female body as the sole mediator between health and disease with both empowering and disempowering consequences for both young men and women. Much like DeTora and Malkowski argue in this collection, vaccine discourses often deny women agency.

Embodiment

For rhetoricians of health and medicine, "embodiment" signals a holistic approach to the medicalization of the body. Embodiment opens new ways of examining assumptions that phallogocentric rhetorical theories cannot easily uncover. Melonçon (2018) argued that RHM research "should place the body 'in direct relations with the flows and particles of other bodies and things' as a way to understand how the body experiences health and illness individually and/or within larger systems" (Grosz, 1994, p. 168; Melonçon, 2018, p. 97). When the human body is perceived as something that is static, it is more easily conceived of as controlled/able by social and cultural discourse. In vaccination discourses, the body is placed in the realm of "diseased" or in a state of disease risk. Lewis (2008) explains that:

> to talk this way implies that the disease is something that can be possessed; that it is, in some way, distinct from the person who "has it." Thus, the disease becomes the identity of the person, distinguishing it as a real and distinct entity with an existence of its own.

(pp. 407–408)

With our social and cultural life experiences situated within male-centered realities, the male body is seen as clean while the female body is viewed as unclean, contaminated, and the "vector for disease or vessels of infection" (Parrott, & Condit, 1996; see also Bivens, Cole, & Koerber, this collection). Concerning HPV, this masculine/feminine dichotomy positions HPV prevention as women's responsibility because women's health is described in messages about vaccines as primarily impacted by this disease.

This dichotomy is apparent and even elevated in the three Gardasil ad campaigns I analyze in this chapter, which gender the responsibility of HPV disproportionately toward women. Women, and especially young girls, are portrayed as dependent on others, helpless, and at times hopeless (Parrott, & Condit, 1996, p. 6), but they are also portrayed as able to maintain their desired healthy status if they receive the HPV vaccine. Moreover, a focus on embodiment reveals how a woman's maternal instinct or motherhood is hailed as the crux of HPV prevention; a mother's worth is even called into question in these ads if they do not follow the directives of these messages.

HPV Vaccine Ad Campaigns

When it was released in 2006, the HPV vaccine was widely considered an important advancement in public health. Through cost-effectiveness analyses, governmental policymakers and other stakeholders initially determined that women should be the primary target audience for the HPV vaccine (Branson, 2012). Early discourses of HPV vaccination all but ignored men. Recently, embracing a herd immunity approach for vaccination protocols, the 2016 "Did You Know—Mom, Dad?" campaign addressed boys and men. Interestingly, a similar trajectory can be seen in the history of the rubella vaccine (Bottiger, & Forsgren, 1997; Ault, & Reisinger, 2007).

While the vaccine is FDA-approved for girls and women ages 9 through to 26 years, the ACIP recommends a two-dose schedule to be initiated at ages 9 through to 14 years for girls and boys and a three-dose schedule for those who initiate the vaccine series at ages 15 through to 26 years (Meites, Kempe, & Markowitz, 2016). Gardasil made this information public through the first "One Less" campaign, which was published in popular magazines and presented in TV and social media ads with messages that directly targeted girls and young women from these age-specific groups. In general, the ads in the "One Less" campaign depict young girls or women smiling and portraying the image of health and wellness. The visual argument, of course, is that to be healthy one needs the HPV vaccine. These messages situate the female body as "at risk of disease," creating an "otherness" of healthy versus non-healthy bodies.

Parents of young girls were also considered by Merck as a target audience for HPV vaccination and ads. The rhetorical tactics played on the fear of HPV linked with cervical cancer and incorporated specific themes geared toward parents of young girls and women including "safeguard your children" or "female empow-erment" (Buttweiler, 2009; Rothman, & Rothman, 2009; Cates et al., 2011). This rhetorical framing emphasized both the influence mothers in particular have on the physical development of their daughters and their responsibility to protect their daughters from HPV. Marketing campaigns draw on the identity of motherhood and rely on "a mother's instinct" to protect her daughter from harm and ensure a healthy future for her daughter, suggesting that every girl is at equal risk of developing cervical cancer (Rothman, & Rothman, 2009).

"One Less"

An image from the "One Less" campaign features a young, smiling, athletic girl—the epitome of perfect health. The slogan "One Less" is represented as the number "1" on the girl's jersey and the word "less" on the ball she has just kicked. The audience is visually instructed to connect the "1" to the word "less," and the girl's body in motion makes a visual argument for taking action against HPV. The ad addresses parents directly with the bold statement: "Your daughter could be 1 less life affected by cervical cancer. Vaccinate her today. Protect her tomorrow." Additionally, a One Less video ad includes the line: "You have hopes and dreams for her future, and they don't include cervical cancer."

The rhetoric of the "One Less" campaign reflects and reinforces the dominant social and cultural discourse about appropriate expectations and behaviors of healthy young girls and the decisions parents should make for the benefit of their daughters. Specifically, mothers, not fathers, are socially, culturally, and morally held responsible for the bodily health of their daughters. Since images of mothers are used in particular, these slogans, catch phrases, and bold statements are designed to persuade mothers into getting their daughters vaccinated.

However, an examination of these ads through the lens of embodiment suggests that the female body is more than the vector for disease. That is, ads for Gardasil medicalize the female body in ways that suggest the necessity of the vaccine to move a woman's body from potentially *at risk of HPV* to *protected from HPV and cervical cancer*. The medicalization of the female body, thus, presents Gardasil as "medical advancement" in ways that erroneously suggest static control of fluid bodily realities such as reproductive health and sexual responsibility. The implication of this medicalization, of course, is that a woman can avoid the stigma related to HPV contraction and transmission for her daughter in one easy step. This discursive medicalization of the HPV vaccine, thus, situates sexual responsi-bility in the female body alone.

A final rhetorical element detectable in "One Less" is military metaphors, which are not uncommon in discourses surrounding cancer (Hilton et al., 2010). "One Less" ads use phrases such as "I want to be one less woman who will *battle* cervical cancer" (Butteweiler, 2009, emphasis added). The use of this type of language anthropomorphizes, or ascribes human behaviors, to HPV itself, which encourages women to take a stand against their adversary—cancer. While the female body may not be immune to the threat of HPV, it can be vaccinated to "fight off" the possibility of this illness.

"Third Time's a Charm"

An examination of a local campaign makes my argument that HPV vaccine campaigns unevenly place responsibility for public health on women even clearer. The "Third Time's a Charm" campaign was implemented in 2011 in Alabama with the support of the Alabama Department of Public Health, the Comprehensive Center Central Program, and the Breast and Cervical Cancer Early Detection Program. In this series of ads, parents and college students are presented with videos, postcards, and poster mailings that express the importance of getting HPV vaccinations (US Cancer Statistics Working Group, 2012). Importantly, the messages in this campaign intentionally "de-emphasize the sexually transmitted disease portion of HPV, and instead place emphasis on HPVs connection to cervical cancer" (US Cancer Statistics Working Group, 2012). This rhetorical framing repositions HPV vaccinations similarly to other recommended childhood vaccinations. Without mentioning HPV as a sexually transmitted disease, the campaign presents facts, healthy images of young girls, and testimonials used to persuade parents of young girls, women, and female college students to get the series of three shots associated with HPV vaccination protocols.

Even when HPV vaccination messages did not downplay or ignore the association of HPV and STIs, they excluded boys; therefore, when they purposefully shifted to discussing HPV as a childhood illness, gender assumptions remained static, and the ads aimed at young women in college still only emphasize cervical cancer as the impending threat against living a healthy life and maintaining a healthy body (Ault & Reisinger, 2007; Bingham et al., 2009; Buttweiler, 2009; Rothman & Rothman, 2009). Leaving unsafe sexual practices and male cancers out of this campaign means that women are still held exclusively responsible for preventing HPV, even though men would seem to have an equal stake, responsibility, and risk of certain cancers. That this illogic has not been much challenged by the public can be explained by dominant cultural norms that allow women's bodies to be considered both objects and effects of scientific medical discourses (Mamo & Fofket, 2009, p. 927). Thus, the notion of the female body, in the public imagination, operates in a perpetual feedback loop that continually reinforces their health experiences as both problem and solution. The packaging of the "Third Time's a Charm" campaign represents the body in this dichotomous state.

This logic is at work in the line, "Ask your doctor about getting vaccinated with the *only* cervical cancer vaccine" (Buttweiler, 2009, emphasis added). The continual emphasis of a cancer that only women get is tantamount to the assertion that the female body in particular is dangerous; it must be controlled via vaccines. This is further exemplified by news coverage routinely indicating that receiving the HPV vaccine is about "protecting against a virus that causes cancer, cancer that kills women, and kills families" (Blevins, 2012). The intent of this campaign is, thus, to equate the word "cancer" with women's death. The message is framed to suggest that women need to get the HPV vaccine for women to live and for families to survive. The explicit use of calling the HPV vaccine a "cervical cancer vaccine"—a move that would seem to sidestep STI realities—reinforces social constructs of female responsibility within the sphere of reproduction. The rhetoric of Gardasil in this campaign signifies the biological imperative for healthy female bodies to survive and conceive so that they might meet societal obligations to become or to continue to be wives and mothers.

"Did You Know—Mom, Dad?"

Finally, the 2016 "Did You Know—Mom, Dad?" campaign continues to frame the human body as a set of parts that is diseased or at risk of disease. Merck's 2016 ad begins with a healthy young adult woman who delivers the below monologue over images that show her as adult, preteen, and as a young child.

> I have cervical cancer from an infection—HPV. Who knew HPV could lead to certain cancers? Who knew that my risk for HPV would increase as I got older? Who knew that there was something that could have helped protect me from HPV when I was 11 or 12, way before I would even be exposed to it? Did you know—Mom, Dad?

In comparison to the 2006 and 2011 campaigns, this ad emphasizes the role of the parent and not only the mother to protect a child from HPV. Additionally, fear tactics are much stronger in this campaign than in its predecessors. Appeals to pathos via guilt and blame are used to highlight the reason for the speaker's increased risk of cervical cancer—parental neglect. There is also a temporal aspect that situates a *kairotic* moment for decision or action on the part of parents. If the parent acts early enough, then the child will not get HPV-related cancers in the future. This line of argument aligns with other discourses on parenting and the importance of taking care now to ensure a healthy future for offspring.

The child's body is presented as a vessel for potential infection and disease. Thus, a logical argument emerges that to be healthy, the child's body needs to have the HPV vaccine. According to Diprose (1994), in such arguments, "the power relation is asymmetrical ... caught within processes of social control," but since the rationale of herd immunity is based on communal welfare of health, "it is impossible for parents to easily remove themselves from this discourse or communicate a different approach to this discourse without drawing condemnation from members of society" (p. 23).

An important change to Merck's campaign in 2016, in contrast to the "One Less" and "Third Time's a Charm" campaigns, is the inclusion of boys and men.

In the female-only versions of this ad, it is generally accepted that HPV leads to cervical cancer with emphasis on parents' responsibility. Yet, in the male version, the threat of penile cancer that can follow HPV, is *not* explicitly stated to reinforce HPV vaccine uptake for parents with sons. Instead, qualifiers are used in HPV vaccine commercials for men, suggesting that parents were not informed of the deleterious impacts of HPV on the male body, "*maybe* they didn't know," "*maybe* my parents didn't know how widespread HPV is," "*maybe* they didn't know I would end up with cancer because of HPV," "*maybe* if they had known that there was a vaccine to help protect me when I was 11 or 12 ... *maybe* my parents just didn't know." It is commonly understood that HPV is harmful to the female body, but not as widely acknowledged, discussed, and accepted in relation to male bodies. HPV vaccine campaigns that emphasize boys' and men's health challenge the idea that HPV prevention is solely a young girl's or woman's problem and, by extension, her mother's responsibility. This shift seems to medicalize all bodies. However, the cultural power that could come with naming the cancer that might affect the male body is sidestepped. That is, women and girls are still slated as potential vectors for a specific cancer while men and boys are not similarly positioned as vectors for taboo cancers, such as penile cancer. This omission is significant as it undoes the gender equality potential of the ad campaign and, in this way, still reinforces female responsibility for HPV prevention.

Conclusion

The dichotomy between male and female responsibility in medical discourses is not new. The unevenness of gender responsibility can be observed across a wide variety of medical and health discourses. Invariably, health and medical messages perpetuate the "convoluted relationships between biology, medicine, body, and culture" (Vardeman-Winter, 2012). The female body is presented through socially constructed ideologies that originate in politics and power. Female embodiment makes it possible to disentangle interconnected cultural constructions that influence how "bodies" are thought about and the roles bodies play in the choices people make in their everyday lives. Cultural narratives, such as those perpetuated in HPV ad campaigns, not only define women's roles in personal and public health, but over-determine them to the exclusion, in this case, of the health of boys and young men.

Like other vaccinations available on the global market today, the HPV vaccine has raised important ethical and cultural questions regarding the autonomy of female bodies in health behaviors and public health decisions, while men remain largely free from such discursive pressures. From the inception of the HPV vaccine ad campaigns, the female body was the locus of prevention, contraction, or spread of HPV. Even the most recent campaigns that include men manage, through the omission of male-specific cancers, to retain the gendered nature of HPV prevention responsibility. It is important to recognize that the medicalization of health decisions and medications such as the HPV vaccine are not gender neutral even when they seem to be. In each of the HPV vaccine campaigns discussed in this chapter, "the female body is constructed through male-centered scientific and reproductive discourse, which defines women in terms of their reproductive organs" (Seigel, 2001) and, thus, reifies the culturally sanctioned role of the female body as mother.

References

Ault, K., & Reisinger, K. (2007). "Programmatic issues in the implementation of an HPV vaccination program to prevent cervical cancer." *International Journal of Infectious Disease*, 11(2), S26–S28.

Bingham, A., Janmohamed, A., Bartolini, R., Creed-Kanashiro, H.M., Katahoire, A.R., Lyazi, I., Menezes, L., Murokora, D., Quy, N.N., & Tsu, V. (2009). "An approach to formative research in HPV vaccine: Introduction planning in low-resource settings." *The Open Vaccine Journal*, 2(1), 1–16.

Blevins, K. (2012). "News coverage of the HPV debate: Where are the women?" *Media Report to Women*, 40(3), 6–16.

Bottiger, M., & Forsgren, M. (1997). "Twenty years' experience of rubella vaccination in Sweden: 10 years of selective vaccination (of 12-year-old girls and of women post-partum) and 13 years of general two-dose vaccination." *Vaccine*, 15(14), 1538–1544.

Branson, C.F. (2012). "'I want to be one less': The rhetoric of choice in Gardasil ads." *The Communication Review*, 15(2), 144–158.

Brown, B., Gabra, M.I., & Pellman, H. (2017). "Reasons for acceptance or refusal of Human Papillomavirus Vaccine in a California pediatric practice." *Papillomavirus Research*, 3, 42–45.

Buttweiler, B.L. (2009). *Because we have the power to choose: A critical analysis of the rhetorical strategies used in Merck's Gardasil campaign* (Master's Thesis). Missoula, MT: University of Montana.

Cates, J.R., Shafer, A., Diehl, S.J., & Deal, A.M. (2011). "Evaluating a county-sponsored social marketing campaign to increase mothers' initiation of HPV vaccine for their pre-teen daughters in a primarily rural area." *Social Marketing Quarterly*, 17(1), 4–26.

Centers for Disease Control and Prevention. (2016). *HPV Vaccine Questions and Answers*. Atlanta, GA: Centers for Disease Control and Prevention and National Cancer Institute.

Diprose, R. (1994). *The bodies of women: Ethics, embodiment and sexual difference*. New York: Routledge.

Grosz, E. (1994). *Volatile bodies: Toward a corporeal feminism*. Bloomington, IN: Indiana University Press.

Holman, D.M., Benard, V., Roland, K.B., Watson, M., Liddon, N., & Stokley, S. (2014). "Barriers to human papillomavirus vaccination among us adolescents: A systematic review of the literature." *JAMA Pediatrics*, 168(1), 76–82.

Hilton, S., Hunt, K., Langan, M., Bedford, H., & Petticrew, M. (2010). "Newsprint media representations of the introduction of the HPV vaccination programme for cervical cancer prevention in the UK (2005–2008)." *Social Science and Medicine*, 70(6), 942–950.

Lewis, S. (2008). "Evolution at the intersection of biology and medicine." In W.R. Trevathan, E.O. Smith & J.J. McKenna (Eds.). *Evolutionary medicine and health new perspectives* (pp. 399–415). New York: Oxford University Press.

Mamo, L., & Fosket, J.R. (2009). "Scripting the body: Pharmaceuticals and the (re)making of menstruation." *Journal of Women in Culture and Society*, 34(4), 925–949.

Melançon, L.K. (2018). "Bringing the body back through performative phenomenology." In L.K. Melançon & J.B. Scott (Eds.). *Methodologies for the rhetoric of health & medicine* (pp. 96–114). New York: Routledge.

Meites, E., Kempe, A., & Markowitz, L.E. (2016). "Use of a 2-dose schedule for the human papillomavirus vaccination—updated recommendations of the advisory committee on immunization practices." *Morbidity and Mortality Weekly Report*, 65(49), 1405–1408.

Parrott, R.L., & Condit, C.M. (Eds.). (1996). *Evaluating women's health messages: A resource book*. Thousand Oaks, CA: Sage.

Rothman, S.M., & Rothman, D.J. (2009). "Marketing HPV vaccine: Implications for adolescent health and medical professionalism." *JAMA*, 302(7), 781–786.

Satterwhite, E., Torrone, E., Meites, E.F., Dunne, R., Mahajan, M.C., et al. (2013). "Sexually transmitted infections among US women and men: Prevalence and incidence estimates, 2008." *Sexually Transmitted Diseases*, 40(3), 187–193.

Seigel, M. (2001). "Exposing the body." *Journal of Advanced Composition*, 21(3): 683–689.

US Cancer Statistics Working Group. (2012). United States cancer statistics: 1999–2008 Incidence and mortality web-based report. Retrieved from www.cdc.gov/cancer/np cr/pdf/uscs_factsheet.pdf

Vardeman-Winter, J. (2012). "Medicalization and teen girls' bodies in the Gardasil cervical cancer vaccine campaign." *Feminist Media Studies*, 12(2), 281–304.

Workowski, K., & Bolan, G. (2015). "Sexually transmitted diseases treatment guidelines." *Morbidity and Mortality Weekly Report*, 64(RR-03), 1–137.

9

"PREGNANT? YOU NEED A FLU SHOT!"

Safety and Danger in Medical Discourses of Maternal Immunization

Lisa M. DeTora and Jennifer A. Malkowski

Introduction

Over the last century, vaccine campaigns have expanded with the stated intention of protecting more groups such as the elderly and healthcare workers, broadening both rhetorical and material practices. Sociologist Deborah Lupton (2012) associates vaccination with general healthcare trends that established an expectation of universal good health and the idea that most, if not all, diseases can be prevented before they emerge. Yet, this narrative has long been contested. Hausman et al. (2014) have observed that, far from producing unequivocally positive rhetorics, the early twentieth century was rife with discourses that questioned the value and safety of vaccines. Immunologist Ross Federman (2014) describes vaccines, once "greatly celebrated" as currently "under fire" (p. 417). Thus, vaccination is a site of both safety and danger. Rhetorics deployed to manage this tension might teach us about the complicated nature of contemporary biocitizenship and how such rhetorics might impact the body politic.

Scholars of the rhetorics of health and medicine (RHM) identify vaccination communication as a site for social, political, and cultural conversations (see, for example, Koerber et al., 2015; Lawrence, Hausman, & Dannenberg, 2014; Scott et al., 2015), as well as professional boundary work (see Scott, 2016). This contested terrain signals a need for what Hausman et al. (2014) called the "rhetorical ecology of vaccination" to be historically articulated (p. 403). We situate the medically and rhetorically complex category of maternal vaccination within the context of immunization as a public and medical discourse, in order to interrogate the performance of gender in public health policy. We argue that the category of maternal immunization must be understood against the recent move in public health discourse to attach gendered language to vaccines as a result of the initial approvals of human papillomavirus (HPV) vaccines for girls and young women, but not boys or young men. Maternal immunization is similarly significant from a rhetorical standpoint, because of a lack of consistency and clarity of this term in the medical literature. By examining this literature and its public health adaptations, we seek to identify the stakes of vaccine discourse as a means of constraining women's health behavior. In so doing, we identify a series of sites whose successful navigation requires rhetorical ingenuity on the part of multiple audiences: healthcare workers, scholars, researchers, and the general public

Vaccination and Pregnancy as Public Discourse

Vaccination came about as a public intervention to protect the common good, and thus it occupies a discursive and epidemiologic intersection between individual persons and the body politic. Koerber et al. (2015) have suggested that vaccination targets the most vulnerable populations, and this circumstance can be traced back to the first vaccination campaigns in nineteenth-century England, which were implemented to control smallpox outbreaks and epidemics that could ravage communities (CDC, 2016a; Heifferon, 2006). Thereafter, new vaccines targeted the military and children, forming a part of the hegemonic and carceral surveillance state that Foucault (1995) describes in *Discipline and Punish*. Variolation, an early form of immunization, was dangerous and inconsistently effective, and the earliest vaccines used live viruses intentionally to impart mild forms of dangerous diseases (CDC, 2016c). Thus, the UK Vaccination Act of 1853 was expected to harm some children, a conscious articulation of danger to individuals intended to promote the safety of the body politic. These early truths inform the rhetoric Hausman et al. (2014) identified as important precursors to current vaccine debates.

Within the US, continuing controversy about vaccines that Federman (2014) describes centers on the "herd immunity" that protects an overall population rather than each individual. This tension represents a shift from political to individual responsibility for protecting nations (Scott et al., 2015). Medically, most vaccines are intended to protect populations or groups; few protect specific individuals (like vaccines required before travel to certain areas). Although vaccines tend to be discussed as a single category, each different vaccination situation bears specific discursive hallmarks that support ideas about protection, responsibility, and social consequences. For instance, vaccines required for college-age students may be associated with certain social judgments around sexual behavior.

The subject of gender-specific immunizations also enters the debate. As Malkowski (2013) has noted, the selective introduction of the HPV vaccine for girls and young women created a gendered discourse of immunization in what had hitherto been a fundamentally gender-neutral rhetorical situation. This discourse continues despite the use of HPV vaccines in young men. As such, HPV vaccine campaigns have been accused of treating medical interventions as a means of encouraging maidenly behaviors rather than health protection (see, for example,

Mara, & Scott, 2010). Similar to the rhetorical situation that surrounds the HPV vaccine, maternal immunization falls into a highly-charged space, particularly in situations where the vaccine is intended to reduce infant morbidity and mortality rather than to protect the mother's health. The social nuance and implications of the discursive hallmarks of gendered vaccination rhetoric suggest a site that, like early vaccination programs aimed at the most vulnerable, shifts the focus of risk and benefit, safety and danger toward particular types of bodies in troubling ways.

Henceforth, our framework for analysis derives from Foucault's (1982) claim that language is a necessary element that distinguishes knowledge from experience because language is necessary as a means of exchanging information. Ironically, the very realm of abjection, the zone of the uninhabitable, is what permits the subject to exist as a person, an entity defined in contrast to the undefinable. Therefore, the existence of persons as subjects depends on adherence to spoken and unspoken regulatory norms, systems of power and control that exert pressures on individuals and society. Regulation, by defining language, can be seen to simultaneously enable and constrain the performance of bodies in and through sex and gender.

The diagnosis of pregnancy in particular, with its high visibility and cultural expectations to launch into a routine of highly regulated medical choices and practices, constrains and enables the performance of bodies in and through sex and gender. As we will explain, a simultaneous enabling and constraining of women's bodies and subjectivities is not simply a two-way street. Pregnant women are restricted in certain ways; and, simultaneously, *all* women—mothers or not—may also become unduly restricted. Our analysis is aimed at restoring women's power to claim or retain positions as independent subjects in public health discourses. We undertake this analysis noting Bazzul's (2016) explanation of the double-edged sword of representing bodies with language: "This is no easy task, as identifying and changing practices by which one comes to find their own identity is much more difficult than it may appear" (p. 10).

Addressing the Public

Public health materials about maternal vaccinations primarily address current immunization schemes. The WHO's (2015) "Maternal immunization research and implementation portfolio" shows that many studies around the globe join the CDC in advocating for pertussis-containing and influenza vaccines. Documentation describing pertussis, or whooping cough, emphasize that this infection can kill young infants (CDC, 2017c; WHO, 2015), presenting a challenge in developed countries that have committed to end infant mortality due to vaccine-preventable illnesses. As direct vaccination of infants takes months to provide protection (CDC, 2017d), pertussis-containing vaccines can be administered to pregnant women. Additionally, influenza or "flu" vaccines provide important benefits to pregnant women (CDC, 2017a). In any given year, influenza causes up to 56,000 deaths and up to 710,000 hospitalizations in the US alone, depending on seasonal strains and the immunological match with the season's vaccination (CDC, 2017b). While pregnancy is the highest risk factor for death from influenza, infants born to women infected with influenza during pregnancy have increased risk for adverse outcomes (Acs et al., 2005). Therefore, the CDC's (2010) ACIP recommendation of flu vaccine for everyone six months of age and older comes with added intensity for pregnant women.

Despite the specificity of recommendations, a "Pregnancy and Vaccination" fact sheet assures pregnant women that a generalized category of "vaccines" will protect them as well as their babies (CDC, 2016b).

> You probably know that when you are pregnant, you share everything with your baby. That means when you get vaccines, you aren't just protecting yourself—you are giving your baby some early protection too. You should get a flu shot and whooping cough vaccine (also called Tdap) during each pregnancy to help protect yourself and your baby.
>
> *(CDC, 2016b)*

Here, the language is intended to be accessible and nonthreatening, as the CDC uses terms like "baby" and "shot" rather than "infant" and "immunization." Pregnant women "probably know" that they "share everything," which simultaneously reinforces the reader's assumed knowledge and the idea that influenza and pertussis-containing vaccines are an important adjunct to pregnancy. The CDC treads carefully when discussing "pregnancy and vaccination," differentiating between the two specific vaccines that should be received during pregnancy and other, undefined immunizations that should be received afterward. Each usage, however, orders the benefits clearly, creating a space where self-protection is shared with the baby, rather than instructing women to obtain vaccines only to protect infants.

Unlike the "Pregnancy and Vaccines" fact sheet, which employs measured and reasonable language that engages readers in a common goal, the CDC (2011) "Toolkit for Prenatal Care Providers" imperatively enjoins patients and providers: "It's urgent for pregnant women to protect their unborn babies and themselves from the flu!" (p. 14). Women are greeted by a headline: "Pregnant? You Need a Flu Shot!" Across infographics and posters intended to be hung on the walls of pre- and postnatal care settings, audiences learn: "Half of pregnant women protect themselves and their babies against flu. Time to bump it up!" Flu-related fact sheets declare that healthcare providers play "a vital role in advising patients on how to protect themselves and their developing babies against many threats, including influenza" (CDC, 2017a). While these sentiments are largely informed by sound science and goodwill, the exclamation points connote urgency and immediacy. Lobbying providers and patients in this way complicates honest conversation, and a bandwagon fallacy obfuscates individualized treatment.

Unlike the "Pregnancy and Vaccines" fact sheet, this language appears to assume that pregnant women should be swayed by pathetic appeals rather than treated as reasonable beings. It is worthy of note that more urgent language is used to encourage women to protect themselves from the risk of death by a disease that may be considered mild in other populations and that the health of "unborn babies" is addressed in this public messaging before the health of the mother.

Returning to the realm of measured language, maternal pertussis vaccination may be articulated into broader models of protection: all adults and children likely to come in contact with young infants should receive a pertussis-containing vaccine to build a protective "cocoon" (CDC, 2017d). On the surface, the cocoon strategy seems to spread responsibility for infant protection; however, closer inspection suggests that this model merely repackages existing vaccination strategies against tetanus and diphtheria with a recommendation for maternal vaccination against pertussis. This articulation hinges on formulation decisions that link the delivery of DTP vaccines. While all infants and young children are recommended to receive the DTP vaccine according to a set schedule, adolescents and adults should receive the Tdap booster every ten years. Tetanus and diphtheria can be fatal to all age groups; thus, the cocoon can be seen as a purely rhetorical practice that groups maternal immunization with existing vaccination recommendations in order to fulfill the promise of vaccines—prevention of all childhood diseases—as well as reinforcing protection for family members against other deadly diseases. Only maternal immunization is novel in this setting.

Collectively, the suite of the CDC's public communications to women and the WHO's portfolio of maternal immunization research and implementation articulate many scientific questions and recommendations using language that can discourage patient-centered agency and prevent the discussions women's health activists have long fought to ensure. Rhetorically ingenious agents seek opportunities to unpack the knowledge claims in these spaces and consider alternative viewpoints. Tellingly, while the general accounting for vaccines in pregnancy treats women like thinking subjects, appealing to their knowledge and reason, posters and infographics about influenza, which is potentially fatal to pregnant women, appeal to emotion and authority. Pregnant women are encouraged to step in line and follow expert advice and trends. The discursive roots of this trend may be traced back to medical science. In the next section, we review the peer-reviewed literature on maternal vaccinations, with an emphasis on top-tier medical journals, which are an important source for the public health documents we just reviewed. In so doing, we identify yet another site requiring rhetorical ingenuity.

Medical Discourses

The medical discourse of maternal vaccination that underpins the public health messages presented above is complicated by poor consistency in its use of terminology, and thus requires a species of rhetorical ingenuity for even general reading. Since a goal of maternal immunization is to prevent disease in newborn infants, the term, by necessity, covers several types of interventions. Saad Omer's (2016) pivotal review in *NEJM*, a gold standard for medical knowledge, begins with the unprotected infant, a rationale that gradually morphs to include pregnant women:

> This vulnerability of infants who are too young to be vaccinated can be addressed by means of maternal vaccination. Moreover, several infections, such as influenza and hepatitis E, are considered to be associated with increased morbidity and mortality during pregnancy. Maternal vaccines, given their potential effect on maternal and infant morbidity and mortality, are the next frontier in vaccinology.

This medical model treats women as corporeal conduits for protecting newborn infants against infection; protecting the pregnant women from increased risks of certain diseases appears to be a secondary consideration. The transposition of maternal and infant in the final sentence suggests a rhetorical move to justify risks to pregnant women. Similar patterns of rhetorical slippage can be seen in an executive summary of a *Lancet Infectious Diseases*, Bill and Melinda Gates-sponsored series on maternal immunization (2017):

> Maternal immunization has the potential to substantially reduce morbidity and mortality from infectious diseases after birth. The success of tetanus, influenza, and pertussis immunization during pregnancy has led to consideration of additional maternal immunization strategies.

The editor renders immunization during pregnancy and the protection of infants from disease into a series of equivalencies. This rhetorical trajectory might be articulated against WHO efforts to end neonatal tetanus, beginning in 1989 with a focus on infants and later expanding to include pregnant women in 2015. In fact, these texts explicitly leverage such prior experience, citing the long history of vaccines to prevent childhood diseases.

Omer hints that consistent terminology in maternal immunization is impeded by scientific, logistical, and immunologic questions. For example, physiologic changes in pregnancy affect immune responses, and different pathogens adversely affect women and newborn infants. Further questions include the timing of vaccines relative to pregnancy and birth (Omer, 2016; WHO, 2015). Thus, medical discourses of immunization toggle between molecular and public health scales, eliding women as thinking agents as opposed to the backdrop for molecular interactions or a population to be managed. This pattern of discourse is evident when reading across *The Lancet* series, WHO materials, and FDA Guidelines. A further problem is the difficulty in justifying the risk to benefit ratio of most investigational maternal vaccine strategies, which require a single vaccine given to the pregnant woman to protect a specific infant (Omer, 2016). The term maternal is used to bracket all of these concerns, leaving the reader to articulate each individual performance as a unique entity.

One reason for the semantic fluidity surrounding maternal vaccination is the weight of past vaccine rhetoric, the decades-long attempt to eliminate childhood diseases. In this narrative, vaccinating pregnant women is mere logistics: newborn infants need time to develop immune responses to vaccines, leaving the mother's body as the only potential source of needed antibodies (see Raya et al., 2017; Heath et al., 2017). Using the same term to describe vaccines intended to protect pregnant women or both women and infants from disease (see Marchant et al., 2017) overburdens semiotic limitations, collapsing these situations, not just rhetorically but materially and creating a space of abjection in which women and infants can no longer be considered as independent subjects. Ivo Vojtek et al. (2018) add the concerns of the fetus to this discourse. It becomes unclear where safety and danger reside because it is impossible to separate, or articulate, these various subjects. Thus, only a rhetorically ingenious and scientifically literate actor has any chance of unpacking this discourse effectively.

Another discursive problem in the medical literature is the conflation of pregnancy, the postpartum period, breastfeeding, or even the possibility of becoming pregnant with maternal vaccination. Pregnancies fail for many reasons, and in countries with high infant and postpartum mortality—a key target for maternal vaccination—this usage is particularly troubling. Medical papers, like Marchant et al.'s (2017) discussion of maternal immunization in low- and middle-income countries, tend to consider pre-term births as a logistical, immunological hurdle. A further material complication in this discussion, as Omer (2016) notes, is that pregnant women receive vaccines not coded as maternal, which raises questions about whether the danger to a fetus (significantly, Omer considers the fetus only in this specific context) supersedes the need to protect an individual woman or her herd cohort. Omer (2016) also observes that the women most likely to undergo immunization without realizing they are pregnant tend to receive the most medically dangerous products, such as yellow fever, rabies, plague, typhus, or cholera vaccines. Women attending the Hajj, which generally requires vaccination against influenza, meningococcal disease, and other diseases depending on country of origin, might also receive vaccines before realizing that they have become pregnant (Omer, 2016). Thus, maternal immunization must be articulated against other settings in which women receive vaccines, and the dangers to women, infants, and even fetuses must be balanced against individual and collective safety.

Obviously, medical discussions of maternal vaccination would benefit from more specific and precise terminologies. In the medical literature, individual authors attempt to work around the problem by defining terms for the purposes of each individual paper. This strategy has a weight of tradition behind it: as Charles Bazerman (1987) and Alan Gross (1990) have noted, the structured scientific format displaces arguments across multiple papers, creating a culture of reading and writing that requires the ongoing articulation of past knowledge into current communication. This mode of rhetorical responsibility requires a type of ingenuity—drawing on post-graduate education and the medical literature—unfamiliar to most general audiences, including many highly educated, but scientifically naïve people. Scientific discourse communities normalize their fragmented discursive practices, making it unlikely that alignment of terminology will occur unless requested by a regulatory body, and thus reinforcing an ongoing need for rhetorical agency and ingenuity in deciphering medical and scientific texts. We anticipate that the biomedical discourse of maternal immunization will remain fluid, potentially incorporating all women, and collapsing their interests and safety into the welfare of young infants, or even in Vojtek et al.'s (2018) discussion, the fetus. Although the medical community may be accustomed to terms that shift meaning slightly from use to use, the general public may have difficulty with such ever-changing semantics. As we discussed, medical information may be presented to the general public in potentially problematic, gendered ways that require another type of ingenuity—one informed by conscious agency as well as science—to decipher.

Conclusion

In *The Vaccine Narrative*, Jacob Heller notes, "Today, vaccines are highly respected and compliance rates hover near all-time highs, despite a steady decline in attitudes towards the health care system" (2008, p. 3). Although this trend holds a host of promising outcomes, the discursive modes used to gain vaccine compliance may cause harm as well as good, especially if unconstructive messages about gender become embedded in what appears to be values-free health communication. Questions about who should undertake what types of risk on behalf of whom punctuate concerns about personhood and agency in a more globalized and bio-technologically savvy world. We aimed to (re)prioritize and situate conversations about pregnancy and vaccination with the material consequences of symbolic subjectification: the abjection of certain people in an attempt to protect others. We found that maternal vaccination, like HPV vaccination, is a site where social constructions of sex, gender, and femininity creep into medical discourse, creating a double-bind for women who seek to behave like thinking subjects. Women might therefore need to act as activist interpreters in these contexts, employing rhetorical ingenuity to achieve the best health outcomes for themselves and the other people for whom they may seek to advocate.

Discourses of vaccination can sanitize and conceal cultural messages about appropriate behavior for women, treat women as a dehumanized sites of public discourse, or insist that women think of others first. While public health agencies and researchers likely are not purposefully creating narratives of self-sacrifice, we observed that certain maternal vaccine discourses lose sight of women in their zeal to save the lives of infants. And both women and infants can become lost in the aim to fulfill the promise of vaccination more generally: the elimination of all infectious disease. It becomes the task of rhetoricians to illuminate the complicated and consequential nature of communication surrounding vaccinations, especially because the myriad articulations of prior and current vaccine rhetorics render language and meaning unstable, calling into question whether the public can find a voice in these settings at all. This is not to say that women or physicians should not act to protect infants, but rather that any rhetoric that elides personal agency undercuts all meaningful health advocacy and therefore requires further examination and, perhaps, negotiation. Rhetorical ingenuity is one means of restoring personal agency in this regard.

Questions about medical advocacy by and for pregnant women and young infants will undoubtedly continue to generate public debate. In the case of maternal vaccination, multiple modes of communication contribute to an overall cultural model of appropriate femininity as self-sacrificing, which ironically can undercut the concerns of both women and infants. Rhetoricians should remain vigilant about unspoken assumptions in public health materials because they can get in the way of their own goals and limit both personal agency and effective healthcare delivery. The most profound possible losses here articulate both material and social registers: a profound sacrifice of personal agency that does nothing to promote enhanced health or safety for anyone. Shifts in perspective will require additional, critical examination of the various rhetorics that contribute to public health discussions more broadly and, in the case of vaccination and pregnancy, the ways that collapsing the concerns of any individual into that of another creates unanticipated dangers. New, rhetorically ingenious ways of advocating for women, as for all people impacted by medical science, then, require astute readings of public health texts as well as the medical literature. Further education and more nuanced public health messages may contribute to the goal of fostering rhetorical ingenuity in the context of maternal immunization.

References

Acs, N., Bánhidy, F., Puhó, E., & Czeizel, A.E. (2005). "Maternal influenza during pregnancy and risk of congenital abnormalities in offspring." *Birth Defects Research Part A: Clinical and Molecular Teratology*, 73(12), 989–996.

Bazerman, C. (1987). "Codifying the social scientific style: the APA publication manual as a behaviorist rhetoric." In J. Nelson, A. Megill & D. McCloskey (Eds.). *The Rhetoric of the Human Sciences* (pp. 125–144). Madison, WI: University of Wisconsin Press.

Bazzul, J. (2016). *Ethics and science education: How subjectivity matters*. New York: Springer.

Centers for Disease Control and Prevention (2010). "Prevention and control of influenza with vaccines: Recommendations of the Advisory Committee on Immunization Practices." Retrieved from www.cdc.gov/mmwr/preview/mmwrhtml/rr5908a1.htm

Centers for Disease Control and Prevention (2011). "Toolkit for prenatal care providers." Retrieved from www.cdc.gov/vaccines/pregnancy/hcp-toolkit/index.html

Centers for Disease Control and Prevention (2016a). "History of smallpox." Retrieved from www.cdc.gov/smallpox/history/history.html

Centers for Disease Control and Prevention (2016b). "Pregnancy and vaccines." Retrieved from www.cdc.gov/vaccines/pregnancy/pregnant-women/index.html

Centers for Disease Control and Prevention (2016c). "The spread and eradication of smallpox." Retrieved from www.cdc.gov/smallpox/history/smallpox-origin.html

Centers for Disease Control and Prevention (2017a). "About flu." Retrieved from www.cdc.gov/flu/about/index.html

Centers for Disease Control and Prevention (2017b). "Disease burden of influenza." Retrieved from www.cdc.gov/flu/about/disease/burden.html

Centers for Disease Control and Prevention (2017c). "Pregnancy and whooping cough." Retrieved from www.cdc.gov/pertussis/pregnant/index.html

Centers for Disease Control and Prevention (2017d). "Surround babies with protection." Retrieved from www.cdc.gov/pertussis/pregnant/mom/protection.html

Federman, R.S. (2014). "Understanding vaccines: A public imperative." *Yale Journal of Biology and Medicine*, 87, 417–422.

Foucault, M. (1982). *The archaeology of knowledge: And the discourse on language.* (A.M. Sheridan Smith, Trans.) New York: Vintage.

Foucault, M. (1995). *Discipline and punish: The birth of the prison.* (A.M. Sheridan Smith, Trans.) New York: Vintage.

Gross, A. (1990). *The rhetoric of science.* Cambridge, MA: Harvard University Press.

Hausman, B.L., Ghebremichael, M., Hayek, P., & Mack, E. (2014). "'Poisonous, filthy, loathsome, damnable stuff': The rhetorical ecology of vaccination concern." *Yale Journal of Biology & Medicine*, 87, 403–416.

Heath, P.T., Culley, F.J., Jones, C.E., Kampmann, B., Le Doare, K., Nunes, M.C., ... & Openshaw, P.J. (2017). "Group B streptococcus and respiratory syncytial virus immunisation during pregnancy: a landscape analysis." *Lancet Infectious Diseases*, 17, e223–e234.

Heifferon, B. (2006). "The new smallpox: An epidemic of words?" *Rhetoric Review*, 25(1), 76–93.

Heller, J. (2008). *The vaccine narrative.* Nashville, TN: Vanderbilt University Press.

Koerber, A. (2006). "Rhetorical agency, resistance, and the disciplinary rhetorics of breastfeeding." *Technical Communication Quarterly*, 15, 87–101.

Koerber, A., Arduser, L., Bennett, J., Kolodziejski, L., & Sastry, S. (2015). "Risk and vulnerable, medicalized bodies." *POROI: An Interdisciplinary Journal of Rhetorical Analysis and Invention*, 11, 1–9.

Lancet, The. "Maternal Immunization Series." (2017). Retrieved from www.thelancet.com/series/maternal-immunisation

Lawrence, H.Y., Hausman, B.L., & Dannenberg, C.J. (2014). "Reframing medicine's publics: The local as a public of vaccine refusal." *Journal of Medical Humanities*, 35, 111–129.

Lupton, D. (2012). *Medicine as culture: Illness, disease and the body in Western societies* (3rd ed.). New York: Sage.

Malkowski, J.A. (2013). "Confessions of a pharmaceutical company: Narrative, voice, and gendered dialectics in the case of Gardasil." *Health Communication*, 29, 81–92.

Mara, M., & Scott, J.B. (2010). "Spreading the (dis)ease: Gardasil and the gendering of HPV." *Feminist Formations*, 22, 124–143.

Marchant, A., Sadarangani, M., Garand, M., Dauby, N., Verhasselt, V., Pereira, L., ... & Kollman, T.R. (2017). "Maternal immunisation: Collaborating with mother nature." *Lancet Infectious Diseases*, 17, e197–e208.

National Institutes of Health. (2011). "History of medicine, visual culture exhibition." Retrieved from www.nlm.nih.gov/exhibition/visualculture/infectious13.html

Omer, S. (2016). "Maternal immunisation." *New England Journal of Medicine*, 367, 1256–1267.

Raya, B.A., Edwards, K.M., Schiefele, D.W., & Halpern, S.A. (2017). "Pertussis and influenza immunisation during pregnancy: A landscape review." *Lancet Infectious Diseases*, 17, e209–e222.

Scott, J.B. (2016). "Boundary work and the construction of scientific authority in the vaccines-autism controversy." *Journal of Technical Writing and Communication*, 46, 59–82.

Scott, J.L., Kondrlik, K.E., Lawrence, H.Y., Popham, S.L., & Welhausen, C. (2015). "Rhetoric, Ebola, and vaccination: A conversation among scholars." *POROI: An Interdisciplinary Journal of Rhetorical Analysis and Invention*, 11, 1–26.

Vojtek, I., Dieussart, I., Doherty, T.M., Franck, V., Hanssens, L., Miller, J., … & Vyse, A. (2018). "Maternal immunization: Where are we now and how to move forward?" *Annals of Medicine*, 50, 193–208.

World Health Organization (2015). "Maternal immunization website and portfolio." Retrieved from www.who.int/immunization/research/development/Portfolio_materna l_immunization_activities.pdf?ua=1

10

"MOST DOCTORS WILL JUST SAY 'STOP RUNNING'"

Women Runners' Narratives, Agency, and Identity

Billie R. Tadros

Introduction

In 2014, I was an avid runner training to meet the qualifying time requirements for the Boston Marathon when I sustained several traumatic knee injuries as a passenger in a car accident, which required two surgical interventions. I suffered ruptures, not just to the anatomy of my knee, but also to my understandings of my identity and embodied self. So, I turned to feminist phenomenology and autoethnography to answer this question: If I couldn't *right* my gendered body, how could I *write* it?

In this essay, I claim that doctors' narratives for injured women runners' diagnoses and prognoses are frequently gendered; these narratives assign these patients limited scripts for recovery that are based on essentialized and culturally reproduced assumptions about the female gender. I argue that such gendered narratives have both material and discursive consequences for injured women runners. I begin by describing the larger study from which this essay derives and defining the role of feminist phenomenology in acknowledging both the materiality and the discursivity of injured women runners' bodies, as well as in distinguishing patients' personal narratives from doctors' medical narratives. I then discuss the ways that cultural conflations of biological sex with gender perpetuate gendered diagnoses and prognoses, and risk disabling patients' textual agency and materially impacting their physical bodies.

I use the term "textual agency" to refer to a subject's narrative command both of language (e.g. through speech, through writing) and of her embodied subjectivity, which together allow her to tell her own story. Textual agency emphasizes the ways that both language and bodies are texts through which subjects speak, interpret, and are themselves interpreted. I follow this discussion by offering an autoethnographic examination of my own experiences of treatment and doctors' narratives for my injury and recovery, as well as analysis of the experiences of other injured women runners—in particular, the experiences of three women whom I interviewed: Jamie, Addison, and Gabby.[1] I conclude by examining some of the ways that women exercise textual agency in seeking medical treatment and by arguing that when women share their personal injury narratives, they provide narrative alternatives to the existing culturally reproduced gendered narratives that so often inform doctors' narratives for injured women runners' diagnosis, treatment, and recovery.

Methods

Between May and August 2016, I collected personal narrative data from 81 self-identified women runners, conducted interviews (in person, via Skype, and over the phone) with 34 of these women, and collected survey responses from 48 of them.[2] Participants met the following inclusion criteria: Each of them identified as a woman and as a runner for at least one year (whether or not she still identified as a runner), had sustained at least one traumatic injury (microtraumatic or macrotraumatic)[3] during that period of time that temporarily or permanently disabled her from running and for which she sought medical treatment, and was or had been training to run at least one race of at least 5 kilometers in distance at the time of her injury or injuries. Criteria were modeled in part on Russell and Wiese-Bjornstal's (2015) study of long-distance runners, though my research departs from theirs in that it focuses specifically on woman-identified runners and specifically on those who sought medical treatment for their injuries.[4] This chapter is based on the data from the first ten interviews and from the 48 completed surveys.[5]

Textual Agency and "Narrative Surrender": Patients' Narratives and Doctors' Narratives

Personal narratives, or "the stories we tell ourselves and others about who we are … are increasingly understood to play a crucial role in the formation of identity," especially stories of trials or traumas, which "are transformed and given meaning" through personal narrative (Mair, 2010, p. 156). The storied body, a palimpsestic ledger of its subject's experience, bears witness *to* and *for* the patient, and other agents who touch our bodies, or write our bodies' histories, also *story* our bodies, contributing their voices to our narratives, both materially and discursively. (My scarred knee, for example, bears traces of the work of three surgeons and represents, in layers of dermis and fibrosis, who I was before and after a motor vehicle accident and each of three knee surgeries.) The consequence of this is that the treatment of the patient "becomes a *circulation of stories*, professional and lay, but not all stories are equal" (Frank, 2013, p. 5). Physicians, like patients, are also narrative agents, and doctors' stories are most often "the one[s] against which others are ultimately judged true or false, useful or not" through the subject's "narrative surrender" (p. 6). The hegemony of doctors' narratives in treatment risks eliding the personal narratives of patients. Feminist phenomenology, though, offers a framework for articulating, synthesizing, and interpreting narratives, and may resist this elision, allowing patients to retain their textual agency.

Modern phenomenology, as runner-researcher Allen-Collinson (2013) explains, "seek[s] to challenge mind/body dualism and also mind/body/world separation" and "examines embodied experiences" of phenomena (p. 3). For example, Allen-Collinson contrasts how phenomenologists and physiologists would approach studying glycogen depletion, what distance runners refer to colloquially as "hitting the wall," the sudden fatigue many marathoners claim to experience around mile twenty of a marathon. She argues that, while a physiologist would aim to "ascertain whether some distinctive, 'objective' process was occurring," a phenomenologist would instead "seek to capture as far as possible the lived meaning of hitting the wall … how it actually feels to experience this phenomenon, irrespective of whether or not 'the wall' exists in any physiological, cellular sense" (2013, p. 6). Narrative research methods are apt for studies of injured runners, allowing researchers to study runners' experiences over time and to "gain a fuller understanding of the unique aspects of these types of injuries that have been underrepresented in the psychology of sport injury literature" (Russell & Wiese-Bjornstal, 2015, p. 161). Additionally, narrative research methods may allow researchers to reclaim and rebuild what has been reduced by modern medical, quantitative methods alone, and to study walls that may not exist physiologically or cellularly, but that *do* exist in lived experience. Such methods have utility for feminist scholarship that seeks to foster textual agency and resist mind-body dualism in studying the liminal space of the body-mind.[6] Moreover, phenomenological narrative research methods that value doctors' narratives and patients' personal narratives as sources of data may promote more holistic and humanistic understandings and models of healthcare.

The Reproduction of Biological Essentialism and Gendered Injury Narratives

Phenomenological narrative research methods may also allow us to more effectively distinguish between the biological and cultural factors and processes that influence the gendered differences between women's and men's embodied experiences, injuries, and treatment by doctors. These differences are perpetuated by gendered diagnoses and prognoses that assume cultural constructions of gender which erroneously rely on essential biological differences between male and female patients. Such assumptions obscure what material biological differences might actually affect the success of treatment for men and women, and doctors may then (re)produce narratives that have both discursive and material consequences for women and their bodies. In so many of the personal narratives injured women runners have shared with me, while the patient has been pressed to prove her symptoms, the doctor has presented an unchecked narrative of diagnosis and prognosis based on gendered assumptions. Biological differences *may* require different treatment for women's and men's injuries, but culturally reproduced gendered differences and diagnoses risk simply reproducing more of the same, particularly if doctors' narratives reproduce them by relying on essentialized fallacies of biological sex.

Seymour (1998) offers one explanation for the consequences of essentialized fallacies of biological sex by illuminating the causal process by which language and narrative not only *discursively* construct bodies, but *materially* impact them:

> Men have been encouraged to extend their bodies to the limit in combat, agriculture, construction, defence and tournaments and contests of all kinds. Muscle action enhances the flow of blood which supplies oxygen and nutrients to the bones, which stimulates bone growth and strength. The critical relationship between ideas and actions makes it difficult to separate social ideas from their embodiment. Ideas about masculinity encourage the kinds of activities that build the musculoskeletal system; the strength and the size of men's musculoskeletal systems encourage assumptions about the kinds of activities men should do. This circularity guarantees the reproduction both of ideas and practices and, more critically, ensures the continuation of the patriarchal gender order and its enshrined inequalities.
>
> *(p. 28)*

Similarly, socially constructed ideas about femininity *discourage* certain activities and encourage assumptions about the kinds of activities women *shouldn't* do, such as distance running,[7] and strength training (which prevents musculoskeletal injuries); the lingering bias against strength training for women may leave women athletes weaker and more susceptible to injury, circularly encouraging assumptions about the kinds of activities in which female and male athletes should and should not participate. This is just one way that essentializing diagnoses as sexed can have negative consequences for women athletes.

Throughout my own treatment I found that doctors' projections for my recovery often constituted gendered narratives, and at times I felt that both my body and my identity as a runner were threatened by these narratives. Dr. H, the surgeon who performed my knee surgery following the car accident in 2014, was confident that I would return to marathon running, and he encouraged me to run a marathon seven months post-op. He assured me that although I would "have to push through some pain" to reacquire my fitness as a distance runner, there was no reason I shouldn't expect to make a full recovery. Consequently, I "pushed through some pain," which I later learned was symptomatic of surgical complications requiring further surgery. Demoralized by my injuries, I found Dr.

H's encouragement empowering, but my belief that pushing through pain was the only way I would regain my body-self was to my own detriment: The complications and the damage the complications caused may have been exacerbated by running, even though that running was pursued under medical advice.

Because Dr. H encouraged me to push through pain, I assumed he took me seriously (i.e., he took me as seriously as he would take a male runner of my age and ability), and I was eager to fulfill the narrative expectations of his masculinized prognosis for me, a version of what Frank (2013) calls the "restitution narrative." All subjects are individual storytellers with "their own unique stories, but they compose these stories by adapting and combining narrative types that culture makes available" (p. 75), and the restitution narrative's "basic storyline" is this: "Yesterday I was healthy, today I'm sick, but tomorrow I'll be healthy again" (p. 77). In the restitution narrative, "the active player is the remedy," not the storyteller (p. 115), and it is the *physician* who has the authority to provide the remedy. The restitution narrative is arguably a masculinized one, both because it privileges toughness and bootstrap ethos and because, in orthopedics especially, it is a narrative that invests the (typically male) physician with authority.[8]

When I began suffering debilitating pain and weakness in my operative leg, I was referred to Dr. M. In stark contrast to Dr. H, within minutes of meeting and examining me, and without looking at my X-rays or MRIs, she summarily asserted that I wouldn't run any more marathons—or that, after two knee surgeries I certainly *shouldn't*, anyway. She told me that I should "consider [myself] more of a 10K girl." Dr. M's assessment furthered the emasculation I had been feeling since the car accident.[9] Dr. M linked my pathology to my sex, emphasizing female athletes' proclivity to valgus stress and knee pathologies. (Similarly, one physical therapist I saw during this time positioned me on a table and showed me my knees' tendency to turn inward, jovially assuring me this was "just the way the good Lord made me.") Research *has* shown that female athletes display greater knee abduction angles than male athletes do, a tendency with a posited relationship to ligament injuries (Ford et al., 2005, p. 127). And there *are* a number of injuries to which female athletes statistically seem to be more susceptible (Shmerling, 2015). One problem evident in my own personal narrative and in those of many of the other women runners who shared their stories with me, though, is that women athletes' diagnoses may be essentialized as consequences of biological sex, despite the reality that medicine "[has] more theories than actual answers" for why such a gendered gap in sports injuries exists (Shmerling, 2015).

As I sobbed in Dr. M's office, I wondered if our conversation and her assessment of my prognosis and athletic future would have differed if I had entered her office as a 27-year-old man, rather than as a 27-year-old woman. She explained that even after just one knee surgery (I had now had two), recovering 85–90% strength in the affected leg was a good result for "football *guys*." She told me that I shouldn't feel bad about plateauing at 60%, that it wasn't my fault. My interpretation was this: As a recreational female athlete (not a football *guy*) who had now had two knee surgeries, I should never have expected to make a full recovery in the first place, though this was the narrative of Dr. H. Though Dr. H's narrative for me was arguably also gendered and damaging to my material body, my interaction with Dr. M disabled my textual agency and supported many of my own internalized assumptions about my femininity and the limitations of being female.[10] What continues to trouble me most is how strongly I reacted against my own femininity in response to Dr. M's assessment, berating myself and apologizing for "crying like a little bitch" as I tried to compose myself on her examination table, grappling with the emasculating pain of injury and of the loss of my identity as a marathoner.

The pain of *not* running motivated most of the women I surveyed to find a doctor who would prioritize helping them run again, many of them, like Anya, citing negative prior experiences: "Most doctors will just say 'stop running.' I changed to find someone who will work with me to be able to go back to running," she said. Several of the participants whom I interviewed shared stories about how their pain was dismissed altogether and about how they perceived that their dismissal was gendered. Hoffman and Tarzian (2001) found that women's pain is more likely to be dismissed than men's, either because of "a general perception that they [women] can put up with more pain and that their pain does not need to be taken as seriously," or because women's symptoms are more likely to be disregarded as "'emotional' or 'psychogenic' and, therefore, 'not real'" (p. 21). Jamie's pain, for example, was dismissed as "not real":

When I was in a car wreck, my lung collapsed ... and again, this is another time I think it *was* because I was a female. The police officer that was on the scene, I told him, "My chest hurts really bad, and my shoulder." ... [H]e just looked at me and acted like—"It's your seatbelt. You're okay. Don't worry about it." ... So, for two days I just kind of dealt with it, and then that night I just couldn't breathe anymore. ... It turns out—they did a chest MRI—my right breast implant ruptured. ... And my lung had partially collapsed. They couldn't believe my oxygen saturation was still close to 90, and I was breathing on my own, with that lung. And they asked, did I do any kind of running? And I said that I did triathlons, and I did do long distance running, and they said that was the only reason I was still breathing as well.

Jamie, a 35-year-old triathlete and half-marathon runner, recognized her pain as "bad pain,"[11] but she deferred to the police officer and his narrative agency when he confidently told her not to "worry about it." Addison, a 28-year-old former triathlete and half-marathon runner, also talked during our interview about her frustrations with narrative agents, men especially, who assume they can read her pain better than she can:

I'm specifically envisioning one guy in physical therapy who—he just looked over and said, "Well, honey, how are you? Are you okay? You look like you're having a really hard time. What did you have done? Did you just have a little scope done?" "No, you motherf*cker! I didn't have a little scope done!" And it's that patronizing, condescending "I know something about your body better than you do" kind of attitude, and so all of those things being interwoven into that, like how that layers in with age and ability and race and gender and everything then mushing all together ... captures different parts of those systems that bring out different responses about that.

The "different parts of those systems" that Addison identifies influence not only fellow patients, but also doctors, to ignore women's pain and to determine that they "know something" about women's bodies "better than [they] do."

Equally troubling as the assumption that women's pain is "not real" or not *as* real or *as* legitimate as men's, are the accounts of women whose doctors did regard their pain as "real" but dismissed their problems as *essentially* female, limiting their recovery narrative possibilities on the basis of sex. Gabby, a 31-year-old former half-marathon runner, shared the essentialized explanations she received for her knee injuries:

> There were probably some comments then, that—women, teenagers, as they grow and their hips widen, put a lot of pressure on their knees. ... I probably just picked that up right away, that that is often the case, as you go from a gangly straight-bodied adolescent to a woman. ... And you're more at risk for injury as a female teenager. I don't have research to back me up on that one, but I'm pretty sure it's true. ... And I guess I would put some of that on being female, just in what my body did, that I wasn't maybe accepting of it or prepared for it, as guys tended to grow up and get stronger and faster, and women, maybe—girls often would grow out and not become great runners, even if you were talented at age fourteen. So I think maybe that's what I was struggling with when I hit nineteen or twenty with eating disorders and struggling against my body being a woman, and wanting to go back and be a bit more streamlined as a woman. And not necessarily ready to accept femininity and all of its bodily facets, if that makes sense.

The authoritative medical narrative Gabby was provided threatened her identity and her desire, as well as her textual agency; if the prognosis for "femininity and all of its bodily facets" was counter to a successful high school and college running career, Gabby "want[ed] to go back" to her "gangly straight-bodied" adolescence and ward off womanhood—and the lack of agency it signified.

Addison told me about how she began to question the hegemony of the medical surety that genders diagnosis:

> I really started to think, more for myself that—"What does it mean that the only orthopedist I've seen is a man who is trained in a particular paradigm?

What would it look like to see someone who is a woman, who has a different specialty?" And so things very much shifted from those first two procedures, which was, "Well, this is what everyone in 'the field' is doing"—"the field" read "male-centered," "male-as-generalizable"—to talking to someone who was able to have a conversation about the ways in which anatomy looks different for a woman-identified body. ... It wasn't about "the field" writ large anymore. It was, "Well, as we're doing more nuanced work in the ways in which anatomy can vary, here are some alternative options."

The more nuanced perspective Addison values is necessary for offering ethical and equitable treatment to both women and men, and more personal narratives might complicate and broaden medical understandings of "'the field' writ large."

Storytelling and Narrative Alternatives

The reasons participants in my study gave for sharing their stories varied, but many said that storytelling was a way of connecting to fellow runners or preventing other runners' suffering. Additionally, most participants reported that hearing or reading other people's stories generally makes them feel better because they know they're not alone. Ashley, a 33-year-old half-marathon runner, saw her participation as akin to her own work as an academic and as vital to the community of injured women runners to which we both belong:

> I like contributing to the store of human knowledge ... especially things that think about gender, narrative, rhetoric, all of that. ... [I]ntersections of health and gender are what I do. It's just—I do them 500 years ago, so I think seeing a project that I could actually participate in that is happening right now that actually has an impact on—women—so it made me want to talk about my injury I think maybe more than I would regularly.

And Addison also indicated she sees ethical value in sharing stories, particularly among women:

> I do feel like it's possible, particularly with other individuals who identify as women, to be able to have that space to talk about the ways in which society places expectations on us—about performance, about aesthetics, about pain, and to really—if anything, to share, such as to create a sense of community.

Toward the end of her essay "Grand Unified Theory of Female Pain," Jamison (2014) makes a kind of call to action—or a call to personal narrative, saying "I want to insist that female pain is still news. It's always news. We've never already heard it" (p. 217). Shelby, a 40-year-old runner who was rehabilitating both an ACL tear and earlier injuries she had sustained as a survivor of sexual assault, echoed this sentiment; she also suggested that women's narratives offer a kind of resistance to the ways their stories have been silenced, elided, or spoken for: "I feel like it's important for women to talk because I feel like we're not supposed to [...] We have to consider how we talk," Shelby conceded, as women's voices are often under great scrutiny, "and I get it. I empathize with that," she said. At the end of our interview, Shelby indicated how exposed she felt having shared her story, suggesting she'd be replaying what she'd said later on and scrutinizing it in her reflection, but she concluded with this: "I will feel sick. And that's okay."

I had the distinct privilege of hearing and reading 81 other injured women runners' stories. They were all news. They all contribute to the "store of knowledge" to which Ashley referred: a store of knowledge that inspires women to challenge the limited scripts for femininity, athleticism, injury, and recovery.

Notes

1 I use pseudonyms for all participants.
2 One participant, Erin, submitted survey responses in addition to completing a Skype interview.
3 Microtraumatic injuries are overuse injuries that develop from repeated microtraumas over time (e.g. shin splints). Macrotraumatic injuries are acute injuries that result from singular traumatic events.
4 Contrastingly, most of the participants in Russell and Wiese-Bjornstal's (2015) study did not seek medical treatment (p. 169).
5 This is an ongoing project, for which I am still transcribing interviews. The youngest women to participate in the study were between the ages of 18 and 20 years old, and the oldest were over 60 years old. The 81 women who participated represented 26 US states and five different countries, and all but four of them identified as white (one identified as Asian, two identified as multiracial, and one identified as Hispanic). Seventy of the women identified as heterosexual, one identified as "90% heterosexual," two identified as homosexual, one identified as queer, four identified as bisexual, and three identified as pansexual. Walton and Butryn (2006), though they are talking about professional sporting and its media coverage, acknowledge that "the distance-running community has been identified as White middle and upper class" (p. 16). Though I did not ask my participants questions about household income or any other specific class markers, the sample of women runners that these participants constitute does seem to support the notion that the sport is a largely white and middle class one.
6 I borrow the term "body-mind" from Addison—one of the women I interviewed. She used this term as a corrective to the notion that inquiry is restricted to the mind: "[I]t's not just the Cartesian 'I think, therefore I am' separation—how do we read ourselves as a unit, as a living breathing organism that is sentient and that includes thought and that also includes bodily experiences, and that those things are all ... intertwined in one being, not just separated out? ... [T]his is a question that I turn over in my mind, in my body, in my body-mind on a regular basis," she told me.
7 In fact, women were once *prohibited* from running marathons because of such constructions and assumptions (Pate, & O'Neill, 2007, p. 94).
8 Despite significant increases in female medical student graduates in general in the last four decades (about half of graduating medical students are now women), orthopedic surgery remains a male-dominant medical specialty (Hill et al., 2013, p. 1814).

9 Almost five years later I continue to resist referring to the accident as "my accident." Ironically, denying ownership of it, refusing to linguistically acknowledge its role in who I have become, continues to feel like a form—albeit, a limited form—of agency.

10 This is something I explore in a blog post I wrote while working on this essay, "Cruciate and Crucial: The Gendered Crux of It," in which I write, "I don't *not* want to be a woman, I explained to my psychologist. I'm never going to be hyperfemi- nine—I never have been—and that's okay. But I do hate that this extended cycle of injury and recovery has made me feel that I can never be *the kind of woman* I want to be—the kind of runner I want to be—*because I'm not a man.*"

11 The women ultramarathon runners that Hanold (2010) interviewed described under- standing pain in levels—discomfort, good pain, and bad pain. I asked all of the partici- pants I interviewed about their relationships to pain, specifically about whether or not they understood and could identify and evaluate pain in levels as Hanold's participants did—good pain and bad pain, or, what I explained as "green light pain," "yellow light pain," and "red light pain."

References

Allen-Collinson, J. (2013). "Narratives of and from a running-woman's body: Feminist phenomenological perspectives on running embodiment." *Leisure Studies Association Newsletter*, 95, 1–19.

Ford, K.R., Myer, G.D., Toms, H.E., & Hewett, T.E. (2005). "Gender differences in the kinematics of unanticipated cutting in young athletes." *Medicine & Science in Sports & Exercise*, 37(1), 124–129.

Frank, A.W. (2013). *The wounded storyteller*. Chicago, IL: University of Chicago Press.

Hanold, M.T. (2010). "Beyond the marathon: (De)construction of female ultrarunning bodies." *Sociology of Sport Journal*, 27(2), 160–177.

Hill, J.F., Yule, A., Zurakowski, D., & Day, C.S. (2013). "Residents' perceptions of sex diversity in orthopaedic surgery." *Journal of Bone and Joint Surgery*, 95(19), e1441–e1446.

Hoffman, D.E., & Tarzian, A.J. (2001). "The girl who cried pain: A bias against women in the treatment of pain." *Journal of Law, Medicine & Ethics*, 29(1), 13–27.

Jamison, L. (2014). *The empathy exams*. Minneapolis, MN: Graywolf Press.

Mair, D. (2010). "Fractured narratives, fractured identities: Cross-cultural challenges to essentialist concepts of gender and sexuality." *Psychology & Sexuality*, 1(2), 156–169.

Pate, R.R., & O'Neill, J.R. (2007). "American women in the marathon." *Sports Medicine*, 37(4–5), 294–298.

Russell, H.C., & Wiese-Bjornstal, D.M. (2015). "Narratives of psychosocial response to microtrauma injury among long-distance runners." *Sports*, 3(3), 159–177.

Seymour, W. (1998). *Remaking the body: Rehabilitation and change*. New York: Routledge.

Shmerling, R.H. (2015). "The gender gap in sports injuries." Retrieved from www.health. harvard.edu/blog/the-gender-gap-in-sports-injuries-201512038708

Tadros, B.R. (2016). "Cruciate and crucial: The gendered crux of it." Retrieved from www.BillieRTadros.com/blog/2016/5/25/cruciate-and-crucia l-the-gendered-crux-of-it

Walton, T.A., & Butryn, T.M. (2006). "Policing the race: US men's distance running and the crisis of whiteness." *Sociology of Sport Journal*, 23(1), 1–28.

SECTION 3

Rhetorics of Advocacy

Focusing on public writing and rhetoric, this section includes chapters about the rhetorical strategies and arguments made by and on behalf of women in terms of their own and others' health and health care.

FIGHTING CANCER FROM EVERY ANGLE

April Cabral

I have always been the type of person who maintains my health, especially by going to doctor when I am supposed to. In December 2015, I made my annual round of doctors' appointments—PCP, OBGYN, dentist—and was given a clean bill of health, although my OBGYN told me she wanted me to schedule my first mammogram right after my 35th birthday, four months later. I remember her saying that a lot of insurance companies made women wait until they are 40 to have a mammogram, but my insurance would cover it sooner. Since I was just told I was perfectly healthy, I figured it was routine, and I scheduled the appointment.

Three short months later, in March 2016, I felt a strange lump in my armpit. At first it felt like a tiny marble. I really had to dig into my armpit to feel it—sometimes it was there, and sometimes it was not. Being so "healthy," I ignored this lump for about a month, when it suddenly became much larger—the size of a golf ball. It was starting to bother me. I called my OBGYN, who told me that I already had a mammogram scheduled for a few weeks later, so I should wait for my appointment. I couldn't wait. Instead, I called the PCP and told them that I wanted to come in and have it looked at.

At this appointment, I was told that I may have cat scratch syndrome ... except that I don't have a cat! The doctor ordered a mammogram for the next day, a Saturday. After explaining to the tech why I was there, she told me I needed more in-depth imaging than the basic mammogram that the PCP had ordered. This annoyed me because I just wanted to get it over with. I cried, which made the tech cry, and she explained that she really wanted me to wait for the better test because the basic mammogram may not pick up a lump in the area of my armpit. I wish I knew then what I was about to deal with because I would have been a bit nicer to that woman. I should have gotten her name to thank her later.

The next week was a whirlwind. Through numerous tests, scans, and biopsies, I was diagnosed with Stage 4 breast cancer; it had already spread to my bones. My spine, hips, pelvis, and sternum all had breast cancer in them. I was officially a Stage 4 Metastatic Breast Cancer patient. How does one go from being perfectly healthy, feeling perfectly healthy, to having Stage 4 INCURABLE cancer?

Now, two and a half years since my diagnosis, I have learned that the majority of women who are living with Stage 4 Metastatic Breast Cancer have similar stories. They go from being healthy and relatively symptom-free to being handed a death sentence with this disease. When I was first diagnosed, the average life-span after diagnosis was three years. Thankfully, even since then, greats strides have been made in research against this disease, and new treatments being created are giving women like me so much hope that we can live with this as a chronic illness for many years.

With the help of my family and friends, I started doing fundraising events and created a team, Cabral's Crusaders, that participates in the Jimmy Fund Walk. Over the past two and a half years, we have raised over $100,000 for research into Metastatic Breast Cancer. I truly believe that this is a great way for everyone to feel that they are helping, and we are fighting MY cancer from every angle.

Because of our efforts, I have become very active with the Jimmy Fund, being named a "walk hero" two years in a row and receiving a "First Time Captain of the Year" award. I also took part in a social media campaign from which my story gained over 250,000 hits. Again, these are all amazing things that I am extremely proud to be a part of; but sometimes it is hard to escape the realities of my cancer when I spend my free time planning events around cancer research fundraising. I spend a good part of my year thinking about these events: What we will do to top last year? What new idea will keep things fresh and exciting? Will I even be here for the next event?

While it is good to keep my mind focused on the positive and the giving back rather than the negatives of the disease, it can all be very exhausting, physically and emotionally. While I love all of the support that comes with these fundraising events, there are times when organizing them and even participating in them is emotionally hard. On one hand, I am there with so much support, doing some-thing amazing for a great cause. But I am also there because I am dying from an incurable disease. I truly believe that the positives of giving back outweigh the negatives. So many people have been brought together for the same cause, and my family and I have been blessed with so much support and true love from our family and friends. This love is the fuel on the fire within me that helps me fight this dreaded disease daily.

11

REFRAMING EFFICIENCY THROUGH USABILITY

The *Code* and Baby-Friendly USA

Oriana Gilson

The *International Code of Marketing of Breastmilk Substances* (WHO, 1981) was passed in a joint conference of the WHO and UNICEF as a response to public outcry directed at formula companies (most notably Nestle) for their unethical product promotion practices—particularly egregious in economically stressed areas of Africa, Asia, and Latin America. Instances of company representatives giving "gifts to health workers and us[ing] sales women dressed as 'nurses' to provide donations of formula and advice to mothers" were well documented (Brady, 2012, p. 529). Publications such as "Commerciogenic Malnutrition" and *The Baby Killer* related the increasing rates of infant mortality, malnutrition, and diarrhea as corporations worked to create demand for their formula products in areas without access to clean water, refrigeration, or proper formula-preparation education (Jeliffe, 1972; Muller, 1974).

The *Code* provided governments with guidelines to restrain and monitor infant formula companies, and it set out more broadly to "improve the health and nutrition of infants and young children" (WHO, 1981, p. 5). The practice and encouragement of breastfeeding is a focus of the *Code*, and on behalf of the WHO and UNICEF, the authors articulate breastfeeding as the "ideal" practice for infant and mother. Yet, the *Code* recognizes multiple entities and practices necessary for ensuring infant health and notes that infant health, inextricably linked to social issues of poverty, education, and social justice and infant morbidity, is tied to unsafe marketing practices of formula companies (WHO, 1981, pp. 10–11). Since its adoption, the *Code* has served as a point of reference for nearly every breastfeeding guideline, policy, and study that has emerged from global organizations engaged in issues of infant nutrition and women's health. In 1990, policymakers from UNICEF and the WHO ratified the *Innocenti Declaration* (UNICEF, 1990), which tasks governments to establish national breastfeeding coordinators and committees, ensure that hospitals and maternity facilities promote and monitor breastfeeding and enact the principles and aims of the *Code*, and enforce breastfeeding-friendly laws at the national level. The BFHI is a joint WHO and UNICEF effort to certify facilities and staff whose policies reflect the tenants of the *Code* and the *Innocenti Declaration*. BFUSA is "[T]he accrediting body and national authority for the BFHI in the United States ... responsible for coordinating and conducting all activities necessary to confer the Baby-Friendly designation and to ensure the widespread adoption of the BFHI in the United States" (BFUSA, 2018a).

In this chapter, I consider rhetorics of efficiency as a frame through which to analyze how the policies and guidelines of BFUSA rhetorically situate certain bodies as bearing responsibility for the public health. BFUSA serves as an example of how the broad, long-term global goals laid out in the *Code* are taken up and implemented on a national level. Bringing together scholarship in the disciplines of feminist theory and disability studies alongside rhetoric and technical communication, I examine rhetorics of efficiency within current BFUSA policy with following goals: 1) make evident the competing and/or divergent research and views relevant to this particular policy, prompted by the belief that making diverging views apparent to users/patients improves informed decision making and, thus, long-term outcomes (Segal, 2005); 2) provide rhetorical space for individual, embodied knowledge and experience of users/patients to be purposely and continuously leveraged alongside that of "experts"; and 3) acknowledge the limitations of rhetorics of "choice" as they can shift attention away from the material impact of societal inequities and embodied realities, instead placing onus or blame on individual users/patients.

Feminist Theories and Disability Studies

Disability studies and feminist scholars point to embodiment as a means of addressing Western societies' long distrust and discomfort with the body. Hayles' (1999) definition distinguishes embodiment as "contextual, enmeshed within the specifics of place, time, physiology, and culture" (p. 196), Johnson et al. (2015) and Wysocki's (2012) descriptions of embodiment suggest it is "both active and passive, felt by us as well as produced by us" (p. 22). Acknowledging that "our bodies inform our way of knowing" and recognizing the "physical body as an entity with its own rhetorical agency," feminist and disability studies scholars disrupt Western reliance on "dualistic thinking in the individual and collective consciousness" to embrace identities that are multifaceted, constantly in flux, and inherently intertwined (Johnson et al., 2015, p. 30; Anzaldúa, 2012, p. 102). Feminist scholarship challenges presumptions of rationality and objectivity that serve to enhance the authority of dominant groups and "discredit the observations and claims of subordinate groups," (Jagger, 2008, p. 385). Feminist scholars such as Bordo (2003) reject rhetorical constructions of the body as "an impediment to objectivity" and instead situate identities as inherently intersectional (p. 5). Valuing consciousnesses and identities that reject normalized social categories to embrace complexity—for instance *la mestiza* (Anzaldúa, 2012; Mohanty, 2003, p. 81) or the "in-between space" (Sandoval, 2000)—these scholars make evident the ineffectiveness of a "single-axis framework[s]" that seeks to situate any one identity "as mutually exclusive of the categories of experience and analysis" (Crenshaw, 2003, p. 23).

Engaging issues of silencing, decolonial, feminist scholars in technical communication Frost and Haas (2017) address how "medical evidence" can silence patients/users, reducing embodied experience into a tangible and measurable norm (p. 9). In their analysis of fetal ultrasounds, the authors propose a "power-diffused rhetoric" (p. 30) that "opens up more spaces and places to talk about a range of experiences, bodies, and communities" (p. 28). I argue that this same type of power-diffused rhetoric is needed within breastfeeding policies. Such a move would not only support a reimagining of (un)anticipated users—opening space for embodied experiences, bodies, and communities previously unacknowledged—but would also provide space for diverging medical evidence to be incorporated and understood as working toward long-term efficiency. This approach moves beyond a singular objective truth that negates the possibility for diverse user voices to weigh in and be recognized. With the aim of making divergent research evident to the user, leveraging users' embodied knowledge, and making apparent the benefits and constraints of "choice" in breastfeeding policies, I draw on feminist rhetorics and disability studies scholars as they situate the rhetorical construction of binaries as both false and materially oppressive; I call on scholars to engage in rhetorical analysis that frames embodiment as always intersectional.

Rhetorics of Efficiency

Concepts of efficiency are rhetorically and culturally situated—emerging from, and resulting in, the values of a society—and ultimately privilege particular bodies, evidence, and practices over others (Frost, 2016; Katz, 1992). I suggest that the rhetorical construction of efficiency (both explicitly and implicitly) in BFUSA policies fail to adequately acknowledge that what is framed as most efficient—for baby, family, and society—relies on a disproportionate investment of time, energy, and self on the part of certain bodies.[1] Rhetorics of efficiency as employed in BFUSA policy reflect a traditional Westernized understanding of efficiency focused on outcomes in relation to expenditure of time, money and energy, and that in turn, devalues embodiment, disregards diverging medical evidence, and disproportionately places onus for the public health on the bodies of women.[2]

Emerging from, and reliant upon, the ideological constructions of normed bodies, rhetorics of efficiency invite individuals and institutions to ignore, deny, or dismiss the embodied experiences of individuals who diverge from the norm as established through societal and policy constructs. As I argue in the following section, BFUSA policies aim to bring bodies into alignment through traditional, patriarchal rhetorics designed to persuade—to intentionally and consciously convert or change another (Foss, & Griffin, 2010, p. 362; Gearhart, 2003, p. 53). In doing so, the policies engage traditional rhetorics of efficiency—promoting a single practice performed by a normative body as objective and good—and explicitly or implicitly ignore or undermine varied embodiments and alternative approaches which are instead framed as jeopardizing the success of policy goals. In response, I propose a shift toward more user-centered design,[3] one informed by the disciplines of feminist rhetorics, disability studies, and technical communication, in which subject experts honor and incorporate user feedback—a practice that, at its best, is grounded in feminist rhetorical practices that value "listening, silence, and mutual respect ... understanding rather than persuasion," and engaging "across boundaries" (Enoch, 2014, p. 10; Royster, & Kirsch, 2012, p. 42).

In proposing user-centered design as a feminist practice, my objective is not to weigh in on breastfeeding debates, but rather to call for a reshaping of breastfeeding policies to focus less on traditional measures of efficiency (conformity, initiation and duration rates, and target numbers), and more on user satisfaction and long-term, foundational goals. As noted above, I use *rhetorics of efficiency* to refer to language and constructs that promote an unquestioning acceptance of a single, identifiable practice as both objective and good, while glossing over or ignoring the negative material impacts that these reductive approaches can have on individual bodies. Usability, in this context, would continue to focus on health outcomes, but would also make room for users' embodied experiences and knowledges to factor into how "experts" plan for and measure successful outcomes.

The long-term, foundational goal of the *Code, Innocenti Declaration,* and BFUSA is ostensibly to improve infant and maternal health, but this far-reaching goal has been overshadowed in current BFUSA policy by short-term, quantitative goals directed at increasing breastfeeding initiation and duration rates. Similarly, BFUSA policies are limited in terms of the bodies and embodiments that are envisioned and addressed as potential users. Shifting to a focus on user satisfaction, I argue, upholds the value of medical and quantitative measurements but also situates the user's knowledge and experience as informing and adding to that value: It leverages varied user embodiments alongside that of medical personnel and policy makers.

Rhetorics of Efficiency as a Framework for Analyzing Breastfeeding Policy and Discourse

In this section, I use rhetorics of efficiency as a framework for analyzing BFUSA policy—particularly the organization's Guidelines and Evaluation Criteria for Hospital and Birthing Center Implementation of the US Baby-Friendly Hospital Initiative. BFUSA is just one of many policies that directly cites the *Code* as the foundation for their breastfeeding policies and guidelines. Thus, my purpose is not to trace the *Code*, but rather to analyze how the policies of one particular organization (and its surrounding discourses) that emerge from the *Code* engage rhetorics of efficiency that:

- ignore or undermine competing and/or nuanced views in order to further an image of the policies and guidelines as grounded in objective fact;
- stress measurable outcomes (for instance, target numbers or set goals) over responsiveness to individual users;
- rely on reductive rhetorics of "choice" that downplay inequities and situational constraints, and instead point to individual motivation or ignorance as the barriers to successful outcomes; and
- hold mothers responsible for individual, infant, and public health.

I argue that BFUSA presents breastfeeding as natural yet requiring medical and administrative oversight, mothers as empowered but uniquely vulnerable, and medical staff as responsive to mothers but driven by objective goals and unquestioned medical evidence. BFUSA policies frame mothers as capable of, and entitled to, individual choice but then undermine this "choice" by repeatedly pointing to the ways in which a mother's infant-feeding practice impacts not just her, but her baby and society as a whole.

BFUSA presents their policies as backed by indisputable medical evidence *and* representative of an inherently natural biological processes. The first of three tenants informing the organization's philosophy states:

> There is no question that breastfeeding is the optimal feeding and caring method for the health of the baby and the mother. An abundance of scientific evidence concludes that mothers and babies who breastfeed experience improved health outcomes and lower risks for certain diseases. Breastfeeding is the natural biological conclusion to pregnancy and an important mechanism in the natural development of the infant.
>
> *(BFUSA, 2018a)*

This statement ignores the considerable body of work that calls into question the extent and scope of beneficial health outcomes directly linked to the practice of breastfeeding versus other indicators (for instance, socioeconomic status or family dietary habits), and reflects what some argue is breastfeeding advocates' tendency to conflate correlation with causation. The latter part of this statement shifts from portraying breastfeeding as a medicalized practice, supported by quantifiable, irrefutable scientific evidence, to the natural, concluding phase of pregnancy itself. BFUSA policy and guideline rhetoric serves to establish constructs of "normal" bodies: noting that "[a]lmost all mothers can breastfeed successfully"; that "breastfeeding is the normal way to feed an infant"; or framing standard breastfeeding policy as designed for "mothers of normal infants" (BFUSA, 2016a). The bodies of mother and infant are, thus, normalized: Breastfeeding is situated as a natural biological event for the mother and a necessary process to ensure the normal and natural development of a child. This line of argument situated individuals who cannot or do not breastfeed—for instance, women who have undergone a mastectomy or are otherwise unable to lactate, adoptive or foster parents, or those who choose not to breastfeed due to material constraints or embodied desires—as abnormal and thus deviant, untrustworthy, or in need of fixing. Such language reflects a model reliant on normative frameworks and rhetorical absolutes (for instance, "there is no question") rather than one that draws on varied embodied knowledges to enhance the usability and inclusivity of the policy.

This critique has been raised by individuals and organizations who have spoken out against the reductive rhetorics and negative material impacts of current BFUSA policies. Yet despite criticism by organizations such as the Fed is Best Foundation—which argues that, among other things, BFUSA policies fail to anticipate or address individual patient's needs or adequately account for the complexities of motherhood and infant care (2018)—BFUSA defends its policies. Countering claims that their policies undermine a mother's ability to choose what is best for her and her infant, BFUSA argues that their policies "*are* designed to be responsive to a mother's choice," but that—"it is expected to be her informed choice" (BFUSA, 2016b). Despite indicating that this decision ultimately resides with the mother, BFUSA policies makes evident that it is the BFUSA certified hospital staff—not the mother—who decide what constitutes an "informed choice." For example, policy guidelines dictate that if a mother indicates a desire to use formula, certified staff are required to "first explore the reasons for this request, address the concerns raised, and educate [the mother] about the possible consequences to the health of her infant and the success of breastfeeding." The underlying message is that a woman in possession of scientific evidence and motherly instincts will choose, or potentially be persuaded, to breastfeed. The policy demands that a mother who strays from standard practice defend her "choice" and convince subject experts (in this case the hospital personnel) of her aptitude to reasonably make said choice.

Within BFUSA policies, then, efficiency is situated not only as what is expedient, but also as what is an objective good as defined within the normative constructs of the policy. Breastfeeding is positioned as the efficient, "good," choice for maternal and infant health, but also for financial, community, and environmental health. BFUSA's "Importance of Breastfeeding" page lists the following five benefits: 1) breastfeeding offers an unmatched beginning for children; 2) mothers who breastfeed are healthier; 3) families who breastfeed save money; 4) communities reap the benefits of breastfeeding; and 5) the environment benefits when babies are breastfed (BFUSA, 2018b). BFUSA policy guidelines (2016a) recurrently position breastfeeding in the following ways:

- as medically superior: "Human milk provides the optimal mix of nutrients and antibodies necessary for each baby to thrive";
- as empowering for women: "[Mothers] are empowered by their ability to provide complete nourishment for their babies"; and
- as environmentally friendly: "Breastfeeding uses none of the tin, paper, plastic, or energy necessary for preparing, packaging, and transporting artificial baby milks. Since there is no waste in breastfeeding, each breastfed baby cuts down on pollution and garbage disposal problems."

Each of these sections engages rhetorics of efficiency, suggesting that there is a series of singular, logical outcomes and experiences that result from the practice of breastfeeding. Of particular note, and thus quoted at length below, are the articulations of benefits to family and community when a woman decides to breastfeed:

Families who Breastfeed Save Money

In addition to the fact that breast milk is free, breastfeeding provides savings on health care costs and related time lost to care for sick children. Because breastfeeding saves money, fathers feel less financial pressure and take pride in knowing they are able to give their babies the very best.

Communities Reap the Benefits of Breastfeeding

Research shows that there is less absenteeism from work among breast-feeding families. Resources used to feed those in need can be stretched further when mothers choose to give their babies the gift of their own milk rather than a costly artificial substitute. Less tax money is required to provide assistance to properly feed children. Families who breastfeed have more money available to purchase goods and services, thereby benefiting the local economy. Research also shows that breastfed babies have higher IQ scores, as well as better brain and nervous system development. When babies are breastfed, both mother and baby are healthier throughout their lives. This translates to lower health care costs and a reduced financial burden on families and third-party payers, as well on community and government medical programs.

(BFUSA, 2016a)

These statements rhetorically situate anyone who decides not to or is unable to breastfeed as complicit in the financial, medical, emotional, and productive wrongs of family and society. The embodied experiences of users are discounted as the efficient functioning of family, community, and nation are prioritized and, the policy insists, either furthered or diminished by breastfeeding decisions.

BFUSA's website and literature further disconnect infant feeding from an embodied choice by citing at length a position paper from the AAFP (2017), which states, "With all of the health advantages of breastfeeding for mothers and children, as well as its economic and ecological impacts, breastfeeding is a public health issue, not merely a lifestyle choice." Citing breastfeeding as a practice that "protects a child against abuse and neglect" and "helps protect the environment because it involves no use of grazing land for cows, no product transportation or packaging, and no waste," the position paper and BFUSA's endorsement of it, clearly shifts breastfeeding into the realm of public health and efficiency. Reinforcing the economic efficiency of breast-feeding, BFUSA's (2016a) Revised Guidelines and Evaluation Criteria note that "[t]he diverse benefits of breastfeeding translate into hundreds of dollars of savings at the family level and billions of dollars at the national level" (p. 6). Presented in this context, breastfeeding is, in essence, a form of control. It is less a reflection of an individual embodied choice than it is an obligation of the responsible citizen: The "choice" reflects the mother's commitment not just to the infant, but to environmental stewardship and the economic and social health of family and community.

BFUSA Guidelines and Evaluation Criteria mandate that in order to receive and maintain the Baby-Friendly designation, hospitals must ensure that "all health staff member who have *any* contact with pregnant women, mothers, and/or infants"—from anesthesiologists to housekeeping staff—are trained to promote "the importance of exclusive breastfeeding" and to "provide evidence-based care" (p. 8). The Guidelines leave little room for interpretation. The first sentence of the Guidelines and Evaluation Criteria Preamble reads: "Human milk provided by direct breastfeeding is the normal way to feed an infant" (p. 5). Such a statement denies the potential for varied practices and bodies to be recognized. Immediately following this statement are clarifications that "scientific evidence overwhelmingly indicates" the superiority of breastfeeding and that "breastfeeding is the single most powerful and well-documented preventative modality available to health care providers to reduce the risk of common causes of infant morbidity" (p. 5). When "normal" behavior is outlined as singular and the medical evidence is framed as "overwhelmingly" clear, staff are left with little freedom to address each situation and patient as complex.

This is not to suggest that BFUSA Guidelines refuse care to those who do not conform. The sixth guideline explains: "The health care delivery environment should be neither restrictive nor punitive and should facilitate informed health care decisions on the part of the mother and her family" (p. 8). Rather, the lack of diverging medical opinions and the need for patients to justify their embodied knowledge and individual choices to personnel (who then must document that this decision was made despite counseling) distance the guidelines from a user-friendly design, focusing instead on measurable outcomes and efficiency. Individual, responsive, and contextualized care becomes a challenge rather than a priority.

Creating New Discursive Space

Koerber (2013) concludes her extensive rhetorical analysis of the shift in breast-feeding policies in the US by suggesting, "Maybe it is possible to create new discursive spaces for knowing and talking about [breastfeeding] in ways that are neither scientific nor cultural, but somewhere between, and containing elements of both" (p. 150). I would like to end by proposing two potential, intersecting, ways forward as we strive to create policies that incorporate the best scientific knowledge available, but that also reflect an understanding that rhetorical discourse is always, already cultural and embodied. The first is to increasingly draw on and learn from the stories as recounted by those *outside of academia*—stories shared in online spaces such as FedIsBest, Black Women Do Breastfeed, or Fearless Formula Feeder that foreground individual, contextualized, complex, embodied experiences with a variety of infant feeding practices and policies. Such work makes evident the complex network of physical, emotional, financial, cultural, and environmental factors that inform individual decisions about infant feeding practices and the deficiency of the normative constructs of current user profiles reflected within current breastfeeding policy and discourse.

Alongside expanded notions of who can and should contribute to breastfeeding scholarship, I propose that RHM scholars rethink how they understand the process for theorizing the usability of breastfeeding policies. Specifically, Gouge's (2017) exploration of *improvisation* as a practice/policy/document "capable of responding to unpredictable and, perhaps, messy details" (p. 431) as well as Dolmage's (2009) concept of bridging universal design, which "provides a means for making difference central" (p. 170) and user-centered design, which prioritizes "feedback from users—the idea that users must be actively involved in the continued redesign of products, interfaces, and spaces" (p. 173) holds potential for crafting breastfeeding policies that are increasingly usable for, and responsive to, differently bodied and embodied users. Disrupting top-down approaches that universalize and/or construct normalized users, usability must be recognized as an always in-process endeavor. Multiple, varied users working in a variety of contexts must be considered essential contributors to the process of making policies increasingly usable. Reframing restrictive rhetorics of efficiency within breastfeeding policies will open space for policy language (and thus effects) to more fully account for the varied embodiments, contexts, and goals of women and mothers.

Notes

1 Current breastfeeding policies place this responsibility on heteronormative cisgender women and their biological offspring.
2 I use the terms "women"/"woman" to reflect the language of the *Code*, BFUSA, and related breastfeeding policies but want to acknowledge the limitations of this term. Rawson (2010) and others have articulated that the term "woman" privileges white, heterosexual, gender-normative, able-bodied identities (p. 46). Though beyond the

scope of this chapter, I recognize the need to further problematize the use of this term throughout BFUSA policy.

3 Although expanded on in the final section of the chapter, I briefly situate user-centered design as that which "requires putting users at the forefront" (Dobrin, Keller, & Weisser, 2010, p. 311) and, if done properly, takes into account diversity within, and between, users.

References

American Association of Family Physicians. (2017). "Family physicians supporting breastfeeding." Retrieved from www.aafp.org/about/policies/all/breastfeeding-support.html

Anzaldúa, G. (2012). *Borderlands/La frontera: The new mestiza.* San Francisco, CA: Aunt Lute Books.

Baby-Friendly USA. (2016a). "Guidelines and evaluation criteria." Retrieved from https:// babyfriendlyusa.org/wp-content/uploads/2018/10/GEC2016_v2-180716.pdf

Baby-Friendly USA. (2016b). "BFUSA response to August 2016 article in JAMA-Pediatrics." (Response to: Bass, J., Gartley, T., & Kleinman, R. "Unintended Consequences of Current Breastfeeding Initiatives", *JAMA Pediatrics*, 170(10), 923–924). Retrieved from www.ba byfriendlyusa.org/news/bfusa-response-to-august-2016-article-in-jama-pediatrics/

Baby-Friendly USA. (2018a) "About us: The baby-friendly hospital initiative." Retrieved from www.babyfriendlyusa.org/about

Baby-Friendly USA. (2018b) "Importance of breastfeeding." Retrieved from www.ba byfriendlyusa.org/about/importance-of-breastfeeding/

Bordo, S. (2003). *Unbearable weight: Feminism, Western culture, and the body.* Berkeley, CA: California University Press.

Brady, J.P. (2012). "Marketing breast milk substitutes: Problems and perils throughout the world." *Archives of Disease in Childhood,* 97(6), 529–532.

Crenshaw, K. (2003). "Demarginalizing the intersection of race and sex: A black feminist critique of antidiscrimination doctrine, feminist theory and antiracist politics." In A.K. Wing (Ed.). *Critical race feminism: A reader* (pp. 23–33). New York: New York University Press.

Dobrin, S.I., Keller, C.J., & Weisser, C.R. (2010). *Technical communication in the twenty-first century.* London: Pearson.

Dolmage, J. (2009). "Disability, usability, universal design." In S.K. Miller-Cochran & R. L. Rodrigo (Eds.). *Rhetorically rethinking usability: Theories, practices, and methodologies.* New York: Hampton Press.

Dolmage, J. (2014). *Disability rhetoric.* Syracuse, NY: Syracuse University Press.

Dolmage, J., & Lewiecki-Wilson, C. (2010). "Refiguring rhetorica: Linking feminist rhetoric and disability studies." In E.E. Schell & K.J. Rawson (Eds.). *Rhetorica in motion: Feminist rhetorical methods & methodologies* (pp. 23–38). Pittsburgh, PA: University of Pittsburgh Press.

Enoch, J. (2014). "Feminist rhetorical studies-past, present, future: An interview with Cheryl Glenn." *Composition Forum,* 29(Spring). Retrieved from http://composi tionforum.com/issue/29/cheryl-glenn-interview.php

Fed Is Best Foundation (2018). "Response to Baby-Friendly USA regarding rates of hyperbilirubinemia among exclusively breastfed newborns." Retrieved from https:// fedisbest.org/2018/08/response-to-baby-friendly-usa-regarding-rates-of-hyperbilir ubinemia-among-exclusively-breastfed-newborns/

Foss, S.K., & Griffin, C.L. (2010). "Beyond persuasion: A proposal for invitational rhetoric." In L. Buchanan & K.J. Ryan (Eds.). *Walking and talking feminist rhetorics: Landmark essays and controversies* (pp. 362–380). Anderson, SC: Parlor Press.

Frost, E.A. (2016). "Apparent feminism as a methodology for technical communication." *Journal of Business & Technical Communication*, 30(1), 3–28.

Frost, E.A. & Haas, A.M. (2017). "Seeing and knowing the womb: A technofeminist reframing of fetal ultrasound toward a decolonization of our bodies." *Computers and Composition*, 43(March), 88–105.

Gearhart, S.M. (2003). "The womanization of rhetoric." In G.E. Kirsch, F.S. Mao, L. Massey, L. Nickoson-Massey, & M.P. Sheridan (Eds.). *Feminism and composition: A critical sourcebook* (pp. 53–60). Boston, MA: Bedford/St. Martin's.

Gouge, C. (2017). "Improving patient discharge communication." *Journal of Technical Writing and Communication*, 47(4), 419–439.

Hayles, N.K. (1999). *How we became posthuman: Virtual bodies in cybernetics, literature, and informatics*. Chicago, IL: Chicago University Press.

Jaggar, A.M. (2008). "Love and knowledge: Emotion in feminist epistemology." In A.M. Jaggar (Ed.). *Just methods: An interdisciplinary feminist reader* (pp. 378–391). Boulder, CO: Paradigm Publishers.

Jeliffe, D.B. (1972). "Commerciogenic malnutrition." *Nutrition Reviews*, 30(9), 199–205.

Johnson, M., Levy, D., Manthey, K., & Novotny, M. (2015). "Embodiment: Embodying feminist rhetorics." *Peitho*, 18(1), 39–44.

Jung, J. (2007). "Textual mainstreaming and rhetorics of accommodation." *Rhetoric Review*, 26(2), 160–178.

Katz, S.B. (1992). "The ethic of expediency: Classical rhetoric, technology, and the Holocaust." *College English*, 25(5), 255–275.

Koerber, A. (2013) *Breast or bottle?: Contemporary controversies in infant-feeding policy and practice*. Columbia, SC: South Carolina University Press.

Mohanty, C. (2003). *Feminism without borders: Decolonizing theory, practicing solidarity*. Durham, NC: Duke University Press.

Muller, M. (1974). *The baby killer: A War on Want investigation into the promotion and sale of powdered baby milks in the Third World*. London: War on Want.

Rawson, K.J. (2010) "Queering feminist rhetorical canonization." In E.E. Schell & K.J. Rawson (Eds.). *Rhetorica in motion: Feminist rhetorical methods and methodologies* (pp. 39–52). Pittsburgh, PA: University of Pittsburgh Press.

Royster, J.J., & Kirsch, G.E. (2012). *Feminist rhetorical practices: New horizons for rhetoric, composition, and literacy studies*. Carbondale, IL: Southern Illinois University Press.

Sandoval, C. (2000). *Methodology of the oppressed*. Minneapolis, MN: University of Minnesota Press.

Segal, J.Z. (2005). *Health and the rhetoric of medicine*. Carbondale, IL: Southern Illinois University Press.

UNICEF (1990). "Innocenti declaration: On the protection, promotion and support of breastfeeding." Retrieved from www.unicef.org/programme/breastfeeding/innocenti.htm

World Health Organization. (1981). "International Code of Marketing of Breastmilk Substances." Retrieved from www.who.int/nutrition/publications/code_english.pdf

Wysocki, A.F. (2012). "Introduction: Into between—on composition in mediation." In K. L. Arola & A.F. Wysocki (Eds.). *composing(media) = composing(embodiment): bodies, technologies, writing, the teaching of writing*, Logan, UT: University Press of Colorado & Utah State University Press.

12

"YOU HAVE TO BE YOUR OWN ADVOCATE"

Patient Self-Advocacy as a Coping Mechanism for Hereditary Breast and Ovarian Cancer Risk

Marleah Dean

I stand close to my mother, my eight-year-old hand nestled in hers, as another cancer story is told. I glance at her breast. I wonder if the cancer is still there—after the surgery that made her chest look flat like my dad's. I wonder if it's a snake, swallowing bits of my 38-year-old mother. I didn't know then the snake would be in me.

Not long after her surgery, my mom starts chemotherapy. I am determined to be involved. My parents let me go to her last treatment. I remember her sitting in a reclining chair, a long tube in her right arm. I wonder: Is the snake drinking this red stuff?

Then, my mom starts "tanning." In the wake of uncertainty, she chose to do radiation. Before her last session, I lay my head on her shoulder, and the snake is there with us—its fangs already sunk into my young chest—waiting. I am BRCA-positive, too.

Years later, while working on my doctorate in health communication—its focus on genetic risk and hereditary cancer—I find out I carry a BRCA2 genetic mutation. The snake, which significantly increases my lifetime risk for developing hereditary breast and ovarian cancer, has awoken, and it is now my turn to make decisions in the wake of uncertainty.

(adapted from Dean, n.d.)

Part of my desire to become a researcher—a BRCA-positive previvor as well—comes from being that uncertain eight-year-old. Women, like me, who test positive for a BRCA2 mutation, have a 69% chance of developing breast cancer during their lifetime and a 17% chance of developing ovarian cancer by age 80 (Kuchenbaecker et al., 2017) in comparison to women in the general population who have a 12% chance of developing breast cancer and a 1.3% chance of developing ovarian cancer during their lifetime (Howlader et al., 2018). Because of these high risks, previvors experience fear and uncertainty (Dagan, & Gil,

2005; DiMillo et al., 2013) and thus must cope with their HBOC risks by making informed health decisions (Dean, & Davidson, 2016).

This chapter examines previvors' self-advocacy efforts after testing positive for the BRCA genetic variant in order to cope with HBOC risk. I draw on interview data with female previvors as well as my own personal experiences. First, I describe the state of health communication research regarding patient activation, patient empowerment, and patient self-advocacy. Second, I explore previvors' self-advocacy efforts as a way to cope with their hereditary cancer risk. Finally, I discuss what other patient groups can learn from previvors' self-advocacy efforts.

Patient Empowerment, Patient Activation, and Patient Self-Advocacy

In recent years, there has been a significant call from both outside and within medicine for patients to actively participate in clinical encounters as well as self-manage their health. Several terms have been used to describe this push, including, but not limited to, patient empowerment (Passalacqua, 2014) and patient activation (Haidet, 2010; Ledford, 2014; Sharf, Haidet, & Kroll, 2005).

Patient empowerment refers to patients' personal goals and autonomous choices in the management of their healthcare. Empowered patients are internally motivated to be critical thinkers and informed decision-makers (Passalacqua, 2014). Patient empowerment is an approach to prevention and treatment in health and healthcare, which demands active verbal and nonverbal communication behaviors within and outside of clinical encounters. A foundational tenet of patient empowerment is that patients are responsible for the effective management of their health. The more active and autonomous patients are in their own healthcare, the more likely it is that they will have favorable health outcomes (Passalacqua, 2014). Patient empowerment is particularly relevant for patients managing chronic and life-threatening diseases such as heart disease, obesity, diabetes, HIV/AIDS, and cancer (Brashers, Haas, & Neidig, 1999; Passalacqua, 2014). Healthcare providers can empower their patients by providing information and resources as well as teaching self-care management skills (Epstein, & Street, 2007; Passalacqua, 2014). A process and effect, patient empowerment has the ability to improve patients' health outcomes and quality of life (Passalacqua, 2014; Street et al., 2005).

Patient activation refers to patients' active participation in clinical encounters in order to negotiate control with healthcare providers regarding healthcare maintenance and decision-making (Haidet, 2010; Ledford, 2014; Sharf, Haidet, & Kroll, 2005). Activated patients proactively seek needed information, ask their healthcare providers questions, participate in prevention and treatment decisions, and know how to navigate the healthcare system (Epstein, & Street, 2007; Ledford, 2014). Activated patients are collaborative partners with their healthcare providers. Indeed, healthcare providers can teach patients self-activation—the ability to represent oneself and advocate for interests and desires (Dean, & Street, 2015; Epstein, & Street, 2007).

Patient self-advocacy is a three-pronged component of patient activation—illness education, assertiveness, and potential for mindful nonadherence. Increased illness education refers to a patient's level of medical knowledge related to their condition or ailment. In other words, an important component for patient self-advocacy includes acquiring information in the efforts to self-educate. Increased assertiveness is a patient's desire to create autonomy, challenge authority, ask questions, and engage in decision-making. Finally, potential for mindful nonadherence refers to a patient's rejection of healthcare treatment and recommendations that fail to meet their personal expectations and wishes (Brashers, & Klingle, 1992). Overall, activated patients are self-advocates who actively seek health information, are comfortable discussing health-related concerns, and assertive when seeking healthcare (Street et al., 2005).

In sum, patient empowerment and patient activation are both rooted in a patient-centered approach to healthcare (Passalacqua, 2014); the key foundational tenet of patient-centered care is shared power between healthcare providers and patients (Duggan, 2014; Epstein, & Street, 2007). For the purpose of this chapter, and given the context of this edited collection, I use the term patient self-advocacy, as I am referring to previvors' overall orientation to creating personal health goals, making autonomous choices, and negotiating control in the management of their healthcare and decision-making (Brashers, & Klingle, 1992; Ledford, 2014; Passalacqua, 2014). Of course, empowerment and activation in the previvor community rely on ingenious rhetorical moves beyond clinical encounters, and such behaviors are the focus of this chapter.

Previvors' Advocacy Efforts for Coping with HBOC

> You make the best decision you can with the information you have at that time.
> Deborah Olson-Dean (my wise mother)

Despite the strong push for active patient participation, little research has explored the extent to which patients engage in such behaviors, particularly beyond clinical encounters (Brashers, Haas, & Neidig, 1999). Previvors are a unique patient population—having not been diagnosed with an illness, yet having to make health decisions based on ambiguous, complex, or unpredictable information about an unknown future event. Previvors must engage in active, empowered behaviors both within and outside of clinical encounters in order to secure their future and maintain a quality of life. Distinct from other patient populations, knowing one's genetic makeup forces previvors to consciously grapple with an unknown future and make informed health decisions. For instance, this increased risk necessitates active monitoring of breasts and ovaries and sometimes the removal of these body parts to prevent the onset of cancer (Friedman, Sutphen, & Steligo, 2012; Hesse-Biber, 2014). Further, BRCA-related cancers are often more aggressive and have a higher rate of recurrence—in comparison to sporadic cancers—which increases the likelihood that previvors will become chronically ill regardless of their vigilance (National Breast Cancer Foundation, 2016).

Below, I describe how previvors' self-advocate as a way to cope with their hereditary cancer risk. Figure 12.1 visually represents these efforts, which consist of interacting with healthcare providers, volunteering, sharing personal stories, and participating in research studies. This model draws on interview data with female previvors as well as my own personal experiences.

As a part of a larger project examining previvors information needs (see Dean et al., 2017), additional qualitative analysis of one-on-one phone interviews with 25 previvors revealed performance of self-advocacy efforts. Participants were recruited through Facebook and Twitter. The majority of participants identified as white, in their 40s, married, educated, and had tested positive for BRCA more than three years before the interview was conducted. In addition, I also draw on my personal experiences as a previvor. Like the participants, I have encountered the need to self-advocate in a variety of ways in order to cope with my HBOC risk.

Advocacy Through Participation

Previvors are advocates by actively participating in clinical encounters; their risks create the occasion for interactions with a variety of healthcare providers including but not limited to genetic counselors, primary care physicians, gynecologists,

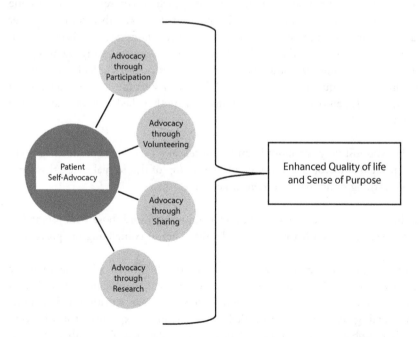

FIGURE 12.1 A model of patient self-advocacy for coping with HBOC risk

oncologists, breast surgeons, plastic surgeons, and dermatologists. With the exception of genetic counselors who are knowledgeable about BRCA genes and offer guidelines on hereditary cancer risk management, most healthcare providers are not knowledgeable about BRCA and hereditary cancer (Dean, & Davidson, 2016; Dean et al., 2017). Therefore, out of necessity, previvors are empowered, active advocates. Previvors must find rhetorically viable ways to seek information, ask questions, direct conversations, solicit recommendations, check guidelines, and know their own bodies. Excerpts from interviews with female previvors reveal their self-advocacy mindset and behaviors.

For example, Tara defines an active patient as: "a self-advocate of your own health." Similarly, Maria said it this way:

> You're your own best advocate and to trust your instinct. It's not easy, especially as a young person to go through all of it because a lot of people don't understand because BRCA is new. You need to find doctors and people that understand not just like the physical things but also like a lot of mental stuff goes into this.

Previvors understand what it takes to be a self-advocate in interactions with healthcare providers. Gabriella stressed, "You have to be your own advocate— that's obviously important—but it's frustrating when you're like 'Hi, it's me again. I have another question.'" She continued to say that sometimes her healthcare providers thought she was being a "hypochondriac or whatever," but she has learned, as Anna put it, "It [is] my responsibility to be my own number one advocate." Similarly, Elizabeth described an interaction she had with a breast specialist when requesting a preventive bilateral mastectomy. When she wanted to preventively remove her breasts because her mother died of breast cancer, she recounted,

> He was just very lax about it, and I just felt like I had to advocate for myself. I needed a doctor that was going to be on top of this to make sure that I got everything done that I needed to get done.

Elizabeth continued to search for providers until she found those who listened to her request, supported her decision, and assisted her in completing the preventive surgery.

Previvors also recognize that they cannot be their own advocate in every clinical encounter. In some cases, they recommend having someone, such as a partner, sibling, parent, or friend, who understands their situation and supports their overall goals to advocate on their behalf. Jennifer explained that, on occasion, her husband served as her advocate when she struggled with getting an answer from her physicians. She described one such encounter:

By the time I saw [the surgeon], I already knew that [the lump] was benign, and when I was talking to her, I kept getting this feeling like "standoffishness" where she was—she was hesitant, reluctant to tell me how she felt about [the lump]. She said, "Well, you're really young. It's not changing." I kept hearing "you've got time to decide" [from the surgeon] until finally, my husband—sometimes he's my advocate—He finally spoke up, and said "if it were you, and you were in [my wife's] shoes, what would you do?" The doctor said, "Oh, I'll have this surgery, no doubt."

Like these women, I also strive to actively participate in my clinical encounters. For me, this means constantly seeking health information from my healthcare providers, the Internet, my social support networks, my family members and friends, or other sources. I request my medical records periodically to review their accuracy or in case I need information while traveling or moving. Reviewing my medical records also ensures that my healthcare organization is following the Patient Bill of Rights (Street, 2003), which ensures the provision of fair and optimum care to all patients. I reflect before and after appointments, often writing down questions I have for my provider, noting symptoms I have experienced, and recording changes in my family's health history. In short, through knowledge and self-reflection, I am able to make informed decisions to better my health, well-being, and quality of life.

Overall, despite healthcare providers' lack of knowledge about BRCA and hereditary cancer (Dean, & Davidson, 2016; Dean et al., 2017), previvors are a strong example of patients who actively participate in clinical encounters with their providers because we see ourselves as medical experts. Tara stated,

The whole concept of [advocacy] coming around right now is a great concept because it helps bring the whole health industry and clients together because there's a lack or a gap [in knowledge]. … So, the doctor throws out some stuff because they have 50 other patients, and the patients' heads are spinning because they are sharing all this news, and they don't know how to take it all in, and so the patient care advocate really helps dive through the [issues].

Many previvors know they need to be knowledgeable and involved, and they are not afraid to seek out healthcare providers with desired traits in order to help them manage their hereditary cancer risk. By advocating for themselves in healthcare interactions, previvors, in turn, hope more healthcare providers will support their active participation and engagement.

Advocacy Through Volunteering

Previvors also demonstrate patient self-advocacy efforts outside the clinical encounter by volunteering for cancer-related, non-profit organizations, primarily for two reasons. First, they volunteer as a way to cope with their own hereditary cancer risk; volunteering provides an existential reason for having a high risk of hereditary cancer. This has been true for me. After learning about my BRCA status, my dad sent me a link to FORCE's website. Never in one place had I found information so relevant to my specific situation: hereditary cancer information, advocacy efforts, research and clinical trial opportunities, and most important to me at that time, support. The few hours I spent on the FORCE website that day convinced me that I wanted to give back to this organization by volunteering. Since 2014, I have served in a multitude of volunteer roles; whether serving as a peer navigator, talking to attendees at an informational booth, introducing a speaker, or participating in a photoshoot for the website, volunteering has provided an outlet—a purpose—which in turn has assisted me in coping with my cancer risk.

Previvors also volunteer because many times receiving positive BRCA genetic test results becomes an integral part of their personal and professional identities (Badal et al., 2018). Cora summarized this when she stated: "This is a part of my life. This is something that I identify with, and I think that I can help other people." Similarly, after learning her BRCA status, Lacy began volunteering for FORCE's hotline. She explained, "It's great. Some weeks, you can get back-to-back calls, but that's been a way to give back and be so supportive." Further, some previvors volunteer because it utilizes their positive test results as well as their own expertise. As someone who used to run medical meetings, Katie volunteered with Bright Pink—a non-profit organization dedicated to educating and empowering younger women about breast and ovarian cancer. She liked working with Bright Pink because it focused on teaching women about good care for their breasts and ovaries as well as educating physicians on how to help patients manage cancer risk. She explained, "So, you become like an ambassador, and you do 'lunch and learns' to different organizations, programs, companies, etc." Given her background, Katie really wanted to know and support Bright Pink's initiatives with doctors.

Finally, previvors feel a need to volunteer because, while there are several organizations to support patients with breast cancer and their families, there are few for individuals affected by HBOC, particularly those at risk for cancer who have not been diagnosed. Thus, previvors are committed to volunteering in order ensure that organizations like FORCE and Bright Pink continue to run.

Advocacy Through Sharing

Previvors advocate by writing and speaking about their own personal experiences. Like volunteering, sharing experiences helps previvors cope with their risk, yet it also raises awareness so others may learn. For example, during National HBOC Week (each year during the last week of September) and National Previvor Day (on the Wednesday of that week), it is common for previvors to post their stories on social media, participate in news interviews, and share in their workplaces. The following previvors' accounts illustrate their commitment to sharing:

> Two weeks ago, today, while it was still October Breast Cancer Awareness [Month] and all that, I did an interview for a local news station about [my hereditary cancer risk]. I am completely transparent about it.
>
> *(Kacee)*

> I did an interview with *Huffington Post*, and it's on the Internet. So, you can Google my name and mastectomy or my name in "Huffington Post Live," and you can watch that interview.
>
> *(Maggie)*

By sharing their stories, previvors hope to make a difference in the public's understanding about HBOC risk and to provide meaning for their own situations—reasons that inspire me as well.

I have shared my personal previvor experiences and research studies about HBOC in two ways. The first is through my blog, "The Patient and the Professor," which I started as a way to translate my research into practice. I have learned over the years—as a patient and a professor—that oftentimes research results take far too long to make it back to their community of study—if they do. Thus, I blog about health communication from the perspectives of both a high-risk cancer patient and of a communication professor who studies genetic risk and patient-provider communication. Since 2015, I have written posts about why health communication is relevant to people's lives, how previvors can effectively communicate with healthcare providers about their concerns, resources for coping with hereditary cancer, and a recent TEDx talk. Each time I present my research at a conference or publish a journal article, I write a brief summary for my blog, so others have access to that information.

Participating in the CDC's (2015) social media campaign "Bring Your Brave" is another example of my advocacy work through sharing. The campaign communicated information about breast cancer risk, prevention strategies, family health history, and survivorship. Their intended audience is women between the ages of 18 and 44 years old since "many young women do not know their risk for breast cancer or ways to manage their risk." Through sharing real patients' stories, other women would not only learn that breast cancer can affect younger generations, but also be inspired to seek additional information regarding their breast cancer risk. My story is one of eight featured women whose lives and families have been affected by breast cancer (see Figure 12.2).

My short video story—like many stories of breast cancer diagnoses in younger women—reveals that my mother's breast cancer was aggressive and hereditary, compounded by significant emotional distress, overwhelming fear, and deep concern for her children. I remember my mom telling me that some cancer stories she

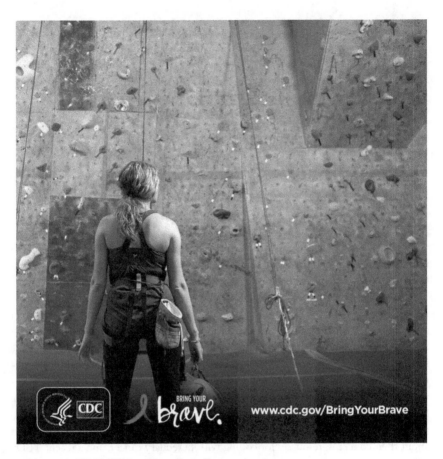

FIGURE 12.2 CDC's "Bring Your Brave" campaign image

heard ravaged her—without happy endings, "It would take days to gather up droplets of fear-covered me splattered all over the floor." Thankfully, my mother has survived. I am lucky to say she was there for my 16th birthday, sporting events and drama productions, prom night, and college graduation. We traveled around the world together. She was at my wedding, doctoral hooding, and she was there when I received my BRCA genetic test results. Although I wish I would have tested negative, learning my family's history of cancer and my genetic risk has enabled me to make informed health decisions to protect myself and secure my future. By sharing my story through opportunities like the CDC's "Bring Your Brave" campaign, I hope to empower others in their health journeys.

My advocacy through sharing is one example of many. Another example in the HBOC community is Amy Byer Shainman, a blogger known as BRCAresponder. According to her website, Shainman is dedicated to education, support, and advocacy. She advocates for those with BRCA and other hereditary cancer syndromes through a variety of social media outlets and her blog. She is a co-creator of #GenCSM (Genetic Cancer Social Media)—a Twitter TweetChat community for individuals interested in hereditary cancer syndromes and genetics—as well as a member of the NSGC's "Digital Ambassador Program" as a social media influencer. Perhaps most impressive about Shainman is her commitment to sharing her family and personal stories and providing information from credible and reliable sources. A look at her recent Twitter feed reveals: 1) a 2018 study published in the *European Journal of Human Genetics*, detailing the current state of the genetic counseling profession from a global perspective; 2) a YouTube video published by the Global Alliance for Genomics and Health about a data sharing platform, BRCA Exchange, which provides information on BRCA genetic variants; and 3) an update on her upcoming memoir. A final example of Shainman's advocacy work includes her role as the executive producer of the documentary, *Pink & Blue: Colors of Hereditary Cancer*, which examines the ways BRCA mutations affect the lives of men and women at an increased risk for developing cancer. All of these demonstrate Shainman's commitment to advocate for change and help others.

Andrea Downing, known on social media and on her blog as the BraveBosom, is also a strong example of advocacy through sharing. Downing started blogging as a hobby in the months leading up to her preventive bilateral mastectomy and continued blogging after the surgery. It provided her with "a sense of purpose"; she wanted to share her own experiences with other people. Downing works to improve clinical screening, treatment, and prevention options for the BRCA community; identifies ways for research institutions and healthcare providers to engage with hereditary cancer patients and the community at large; and improves health care through connections with individuals, technology, and design. Defining herself as a "BRCActivist," another way she advocated for those in BRCA and HBOC communities was by sharing her story on the Supreme Court's steps while arguments were heard for the *Association of Molecular Pathology v. Myriad Genetics* case, the result of which was the Supreme Court overturning the right to patent human DNA.

On the whole, one previvor (Janelle) perfectly summarized her approach to sharing her story with others when she expressed,

> People have told me, "You're such an activist." I don't think of myself that way but to become an advocate—an awareness person for this—because this topic that is very near and dear to me, and I also feel that it's a tribute to my mom. If I can prevent it, I always say, if I can change the trajectory of one person's life or one family, so that they don't have to go through what we went through. If there is a BRCA mutation in the family that people find out about it before somebody dies—because that's basically is what happened to us that we didn't find out until somebody died—If I can change that in one person or in one family, I will have done some good in the world.

Advocacy Through Research

Finally, previvors are advocates as they engage in clinical research to improve health outcomes and experiences. Previvors believe that participating in research is the only way to improve clinical evidence in order to provide better recommendations and improve outcomes. One example is the ABOUT Patient-Powered Research Network established through the PCORI in 2014 as a collaboration between researchers at FORCE, University of South Florida, and the Michigan Department of Health and Human Services. The ABOUT Network gathers and examines real patients' experiences in order to empower them in their health decision-making, provide recommendations for clinical care, and ultimately, improve health outcomes.

The ABOUT Network is unique because it is patient-driven. In contrast to traditional research where researchers choose the topics, write the goals, conduct the analyses, and publish the results in academic journals, the ABOUT Network asks patients affected by HBOC what information they would like to know and what studies would be helpful to improve their quality of life and overall care (Armstrong et al., 2015).

Soon after testing BRCA positive, I joined the ABOUT Network registry as a patient. Being a part of this network reminded me that without research participants, previvors would never have learned the connection between genetics and cancer risk, and advanced technologies for cancer prevention, screening, treatment, or family planning would not exist. Not long after joining the registry, I was invited to serve on ABOUT's patient-led Steering Committee to use my expertise in health communication to motivate others to join the network. In this capacity, I had the privilege of interacting with other women and men who have chosen to contribute and guide research. My experience on this committee revealed that previvors believe they are medical experts who hold key information that can help improve patient health outcomes. They believe each individual has something to offer their community. I now serve on the Executive Committee using my expertise as a researcher to ensure its success. My participation in this committee has inspired me to continue to engage in community-based participatory research.

In sum, previvors' advocacy reveals a commitment to improving one's own health experiences and decision goals as well as contributing to others' wellbeing. Previvors manage their HBOC risks through advocacy in clinical encounters, volunteer work, by sharing stories, and through research participation (Gruman et al., 2010; Rauscher, & Dean, 2017), enhancing their quality of life and sense of purpose. As such, previvors provide an example for other patient groups regarding engagement and advocacy efforts in clinical encounters.

Learning from Previvors' Self-Advocacy

Previvors' self-advocacy efforts offer two helpful strategies other patient groups can utilize when seeking to cope with their own health issues and diseases. The first strategy is actively participating and communicating in clinical encounters with healthcare providers. This includes asking questions and checking understanding (Epstein, & Street, 2007; Sharf, Haidet, & Kroll, 2005; Sparks, & Villagran, 2010). Research on patient-provider interactions reveals that patients often do not participate in medical dialogues because they are fearful, anxious and/or embarrassed, do not understand, are discouraged by the provider's communication style, and believe it is appropriate to be passive (Robinson, 2003; Judson, Detsky, & Press, 2013). However, patients are more satisfied with their clinical encounters and are more likely to remember (and follow) their healthcare providers' treatment recommendations when they ask questions (Dillon, 2012; Sharf, Haidet, & Kroll, 2005). One way to address these fears is to write down questions prior to attending an appointment. Then, at the beginning of the appointment, patients can tell their provider they have questions they need answered at some point. After asking questions, it is equally important to check one's understanding of the provided information and recommendations. Patients can check understanding throughout the appointment, but especially at the end. Research notes that many times patients become overwhelmed by the amount of complex information given in consultations (Epstein, & Street, 2007); before leaving an appointment, patients can comment something like, "Based on my appointment today, these are the things I need to do ... Is that correct?" Asking questions and checking understanding may ensure patients and healthcare providers work together to achieve patients' goals and make informed health decisions (Epstein, & Street, 2007).

A second helpful strategy for both at-risk patient groups and those with chronic conditions is participating in research.[1] Patients can engage in research as partners and as members of the research team (Selker, & Wilkins, 2017). One example of patients involved in research, as noted above, is the ABOUT Network. Research conducted by the ABOUT Network is "patient-powered"—meaning patients affected by HBOC do the following: a) provide research ideas, b) help decide what research topics are important to the community at large, c) participate in designing research studies, d) participate in those research studies, and e) help share the research findings with the HBOC community and general public. This research approach engages patients from development to the dissemination of results (Armstrong et al., 2015) and is beneficial for all parties. By engaging in research, patients benefit as they help guide research inquires to ensure translatability; researchers benefit as patients are more likely to enroll and remain in clinical studies; and healthcare providers benefit as the results translate better to clinical practice and care (Domecq et al., 2014). Finally, patient engagement in research assists in disseminating research results to the relevant community in relatable and understandable ways (Swartz et al., 2004).

Conclusion

Overall, my journey has been an emotional one, but it has made me strong. There are days I worry that I will be diagnosed with cancer. Yet, learning my BRCA status has been empowering, and through my research and volunteer work I get to meet and interact with women and men who encourage and inspire me daily. Although I have a family history and a genetic predisposition to cancer, this doesn't mean I cannot live ... and live well. And, for me, living well means embracing this part of my identity, striving to help others while constantly challenging myself. I do not have to let my past, or my family's past, dictate my future. I come from a family of survivors, and I always remember my mother's wise words: "You make the best decision you can with the information that you have at that time."

Note

1   For systematic reviews on patient and stakeholder engagement in research see Concannon et al. (2014), Shippee et al. (2015), and Domecq et al. (2014).

References

Armstrong, J., Toscano, M., Kotchko, N., Friedman, S., Schwartz, M.D., Virgo, K.S., ... & Casares, C. (2015). "American BRCA outcomes and utilization of testing (ABOUT) study: A pragmatic research model that incorporates personalized medicine/patient-centered outcomes in a real world setting." *Journal of Genetic Counseling*, 24(1), 18–28.

Badal, H.J., Ross, A.A., Scherr, C.L., Dean, M., & Clements, M. (2018). "Previving: How unaffected women with a BRCA1/2 mutation define and construct identity." (Paper competitively selected by the Health Communication Division). Oral presentation at the International Communication Association, Prague, Czech Republic (May, 24–28).

Brashers, D.E., Haas, S.M., & Neidig, J.L. (1999). "The patient self-advocacy scale: Measuring patient involvement in health care decision-making interactions." *Health Communication*, 11(2), 97–121.

Brashers, D.E., & Klingle, R.S. (1992). "The influence of activism on physician–patient communication." Paper presented at the Speech Communication Association Annual Meeting. Chicago, IL (October, 29).

Centers for Disease Control and Prevention. (2015). "About the campaign 'Bring your brave.' Breast cancer in young women." Retrieved from www.cdc.gov/cancer/breast/young_women/bringyourbrave/about.htm

Concannon, T.W., Fuster, M., Saunders, T., Patel, K., Wong, J.B., Leslie, L.K., & Lau, J. (2014). "A systematic review of stakeholder engagement in comparative effectiveness and patient-centered outcomes research." *Journal of General Internal Medicine*, 29(2), 1692–1701.

Dagan, E., & Gil, S. (2005). "BRCA1/2 mutation carriers: Psychological distress and ways of coping." *Journal of Psychosocial Oncology*, 22(3), 93–106.

Dean, M. (n.d.). "Faces of breast cancer: Marleah Dean Kruzel from College Station, Tex." *The New York Times*. Retrieved from www.nytimes.com/interactive/projects/well/breast-cancer-stories/stories/641

Dean, M., & Davidson, L. (2016). "Previvors' uncertainty management strategies for hereditary breast and ovarian cancer." *Health Communication*, 33(2), 122–130.

Dean, M., & Street, R.L., Jr. (2015). "Managing uncertainty in clinical encounters." In B. Spitzberg & A. Hannawa (Eds.). *Handbook of communication competence* (pp. 477–501). Berlin, Germany and Boston, MA: De Gruyter Mouton.

Dean, M., Scherr, C.L., Clements, M., Koruo, R., Martinez, J., & Ross, A. (2017). "'When information is not enough': A model for understanding BRCA-positive pre-vivors' information needs regarding hereditary breast and ovarian cancer risk." *Patient Education & Counseling*, 100(9), 1738–1743.

Dillon, P.J. (2012). "Assessing the influence of patient participation in primary care medical interviews on recall of treatment recommendations." *Health Communication*, 27(1), 58–65.

DiMillo, J., Samson, A., Thériault, A., Lowry, S., Corsini, L., Verma, S., & Tomiak, E. (2013). "Living with the BRCA genetic mutation: An uncertain conclusion to an unending process." *Psychology, Health & Medicine*, 18(2), 125–134.

Domecq, J.P., Prutsky, G., Elraiyah, T., Wang, Z., Nabhan, M., Shippee, N., ... & Erwin, P. (2014). "Patient engagement in research: A systematic review." *BMC Health Services Research*, 14(1), 89–98.

Duggan, A. (2014). "Patient and relationship-centered communication and medicine." In T. L. Thompson (Ed.). *SAGE encyclopedia of health communication* (pp. 1029–1032). Thousand Oaks, CA: Sage.

Epstein, R., & Street, R.L., Jr. (2007). *Patient-centered communication in cancer care: Promoting healing and reducing suffering* (NIH Publication No. 07e6225). Bethesda, MD: National Cancer Institute.

Friedman, S., Sutphen, R., & Steligo, K. (2012). *Confronting hereditary breast and ovarian cancer: Identify your risk, understand your options, change your destiny.* New York: John Hopkins University Press.

Gruman, M., Homes Rovner, M.E., French, D., Jeffress, S., Sofaer, D., Shaller, D., Prager, D.J. (2010). "From patient education to patient engagement: Implications for the field of patient education." *Patient Education & Counseling*, 78(3), 350–356.

Haidet, P. (2010). "No longer silent: On becoming an active patient." *Health Communication*, 25(2), 195–197.

Hesse-Biber, S. (2014). "The genetic testing experience of BRCA-positive women: Deciding between surveillance and surgery." *Qualitative Health Research*, 24(6), 773–789.

Howlader, N., Noone, A.M., Krapcho, M., Miller, D., Bishop, K., Kosary, C.L., ... & Cronin, K.A. (2018). "SEER cancer statistics review (CSR) 1975–2014." Bethesda, MD: National Cancer Institute. Retrieved from: https://seer.cancer.gov/csr/1975_2014.

Judson, T.J., Detsky, A.S., & Press, M.J. (2013). "Encouraging patients to ask questions: How to overcome 'white-coat silence'." *JAMA*, 309(22), 2325–2326.

Kuchenbaecker, K.B., Hopper, J.L., Barnes, D.R., Phillips, K.A., Mooij, T.M., Roos-Blom, M.J., ... & Olsson, H. (2017). "Risks of breast, ovarian, and contralateral breast cancer for BRCA1 and BRCA2 mutation carriers." *Journal of the American Medical Association*, 317(23), 2402–2416.

Ledford, C.J.W. (2014). "Patient activation." In T.L. Thompson (Ed.), *SAGE encyclopedia of health communication* (pp. 1027–1028). Thousand Oaks, CA: Sage.

National Breast Cancer Foundation. (2016). "BRCA: The breast cancer gene." Retrieved from https://www.nationalbreastcancer.org/what-is-brca

Passalacqua, S.A. (2014). "Patient empowerment." In T.L. Thompson (Ed.), *SAGE encyclopedia of health communication* (pp. 1034–1036). Thousand Oaks, CA: Sage.

Rauscher, E.A., & Dean, M. (2017). "'I've just never gotten around to doing it': Men's approaches to managing BRCA-related cancer risks." *Patient Education & Counseling*, 101(2), 340–345.

Robinson, J.D. (2003). "An interactional structure of medical activities during acute visits and its implications for patients' participation." *Health Communication*, 15(1), 27–58.

Selker, H.P., & Wilkins, C.H. (2017). "From community engagement, to community-engaged research, to broadly engaged team science." *Journal of Clinical and Translational Science*, 1(1), 5–6.

Sharf, B.F., Haidet, P., & Kroll, T.L. (2005). "'I want you to put me in the grave with all my limbs': The meaning of active health participation." In E.B. Ray (Ed.). *Health communication in practice: A case study approach* (2nd ed., pp. 39–51). Mahwah, NJ: Lawrence Erlbaum Associates.

Shippee, N.D., Domecq Garces, J.P., Prutsky Lopez, G.J., Wang, Z., Elraiyah, T.A., Nabhan, M., … & Erwin, P.J. (2015). "Patient and service user engagement in research: A systematic review and synthesized framework." *Health Expectations*, 18(5), 1151–1166.

Sparks, L., & Villagran, M. (2010). *Patient and provider interaction: A global health communication perspective*. Malden, MA: Polity Press.

Street, R.L., Jr. (2003). "Communication in medical encounters: An ecological perspective." In T.L. Thompson, R. Parrott, & J. Nussbaum (Eds.). *The Routledge handbook of health communication* (pp. 77–104). New York: Routledge.

Street, R.L., Jr.Gordon, H.S., Ward, M.M., Krupat, E., & Kravitz, R.L. (2005). "Patient participation in medical consultations: Why some patients are more involved than others." *Medical Care*, 43(10), 960–969.

Swartz, L.J., Callahan, K.A., Butz, A.M., Rand, C.S., Kanchanaraksa, S., Diette, G.B., … & Eggleston, P.A. (2004). "Methods and issues in conducting a community-based environmental randomized trial." *Environmental Research*, 95(2), 156–165.

13

ACTIVISM BY ACCURACY

Women's Health and Hormonal Birth Control

Kristin Marie Bivens, Kirsti Cole, and Amy Koerber

When the term *hormone* was coined in a 1905 Royal Society lecture by British physician Ernest Henry Starling, medical discourse on reproductive hormones suggested that experts were intent on discovering the "female sex hormone" so that women could be better understood (Koerber, 2018). The goal of much of this early research was to control women's bodies so that they would behave more like men's bodies, without all of the natural hormonal flux and change that was already known to characterize female reproduction. In fact, this discourse indicates that medical practitioners were intent on sanitizing women's bodies— cleaning up reproductive processes, including menses and hormonal fluctuations and, thus, figuring out how to regularize women's bodies.

Rhetorical-historical analysis of this early medical discourse establishes that curing women of their "feminineness" (Frank, 1929, Foreword), or of the inherent problem of being female, was a motivating force behind the initial development of birth control technologies. As expressed by one of the leading early twentieth-century researchers in this area, the "difficult, time-consuming, and expensive" quest sought to "relieve many of the ills from which women now suffer" (Frank, 1929, Foreword). In addition, early scientists and physicians "groping in the wrong direction and pursuing fruitless leads into blind alleys" (Frank, 1929, Foreword) characterize females' physical and mental health problems as fundamental to society's problems. They assumed that if they could "fix" women, they could also fix society.

In this chapter, we analyze how female hormones and hormonal cycles are problematically constructed and distorted as static and medically interchangeable by medical practitioners. We demonstrate that in today's dominant medical discourses, HBC is fulfilling its original purpose—to control and sanitize women's bodies (and hormones). We argue that current, dominant medical discourses perpetuate a powerful *doxa* regarding HBC, and they accomplish this by omitting key facts about *how* HBC prevents pregnancy and the hormonal effect this kind of birth control has on women's bodies. We argue that these purposeful omissions are exposed in CAM counter-discourses.

More specifically, with the historical discoveries of the early twentieth century as a backdrop, this chapter analyzes twenty-first-century advertisements for HBC, exposing the ways these texts deliver on the promises made in early gynecological texts. We now have HBC that is advertised as having the potential to "cure" acne, take away the menstrual period, reduce menstrual pain, and even prevent certain kinds of cancer. And, in certain instances, HBC does work in these capacities. However, as alternative and naturopathic medical practitioners argue, the *doxa* HBC discourses create and circulate prevent women from accessing accurate health information. Part of the exigency in early twentieth-century discourses on female hormones was the pressing concern that women needed to be relieved from menstruation and hormonal fluctuations with their bleeding, bloating, menstrual pain, and pregnancy—by discovery and application of the hormones that made them that way. We recognize that these discourses serve to reinforce heteronormative paradigms of biological essentialism, but we focus on the ways in which medical discourses define women through chemical hormones in order to unpack continuing medicalized reification of such sex-gender essentialist binaries.

To do so, we interrogate contemporary biomedical *doxa* surrounding HBC, women's bodies, and healthcare. *Doxas* are defined as "commonsense beliefs" that can underlie popular and expert discourses on health-related subjects. Often implied, *doxas* easily go unnoticed because they are so widely shared among members of a given audience (Gibbons, 2014, p. 427). Our particular focus is the *doxa* around HBC that prioritizes expediency and effectiveness of preventing pregnancy over hormonal, physiological health. We suggest that alternative medical and naturopathic arguments and texts provide a powerful counter-discourse capable of productively disrupting the *doxa* about HBC; this accurate information on hormonal health might empower patients by providing them with increased and more accurate information about their bodies and the potential consequences of taking HBC.

By juxtaposing contemporary birth control advertisements for HBC methods, including Yaz and Mirena, with naturopathic and CAM discourses about women's hormones by key advocates Weschler (2015) and Briden (n.d.), we argue that more accurate information about HBC and patient agency from alternative medical practitioners is a powerful form of activism—activism by accuracy.

As noted by Gibbons (2014), "Like an ocean's undertow, doxa can be a forceful current, doing powerful inventional work beneath the surface of discourse" (p. 428). *Doxa*, thus, accounts for how and why contemporary biomedical discourses of HBC, in many ways, fulfill the promise made by early twentieth-century medical practitioners who believed they could eventually fix women by curing them of their femaleness. Therefore, examining the *doxa* that exist beneath the surface of current medical discourses on HBC exposes how these historical beliefs persist.

Doxa and Feminist Rhetorical-Historical Research

Our feminist rhetorical methods are informed by Altman (1988), Bizzell (2000), and Royster and Kirsch (2012), which, taken together, open space in which women's experiences, discourses, and contents can be understood as not only integral to but formative of our research practices. Woods (2012) argued that "an intersectional approach to rhetorical history should be concerned with shifting webs of relationships rather than singular articulations of identity in historical contexts" (p. 79). Drawing from these methodologies, we look at the ways in which biomedical *doxas* seek to flatten women's bodies and embodied experiences into that singular articulation of identity—the identity articulated by white, male scientists at the turn of the previous century. *Doxa*, of course, coincides with the rhetorical concept of *enthymeme*, or "any aspect of an argument whose omission makes the argument seem compelling or intriguing or novel and, at the same time, makes its audience feel comfortable or satisfied" (Koerber, 2018, p. 158). We suggest the challenge for rhetorically ingenious women's health activism includes interrogating sources of biomedical *doxas* about HBC and other substances that are most commonly thought to provide benefit, not harm, to the women who ingest them.

According to Amossy (2002), *doxa* is a concept inherited from ancient Greek rhetoric that "appears under various guises, such as public opinion, verisimilitude, commonsense knowledge, commonplace, *idée reçue*, stereotype, cliché" (p. 369). Crowley (2006) understood *doxa* as "assertions about the way things are—what exists, what human nature is, how the world operates" that become "consonant with reality" (pp. 67, 69). Of consequence, Amossy further explained a noteworthy Aristotelian distinction: *endoxa* is "what appears manifest and true to all, or to most of the people, or to the wise," reliant on consensus (p. 371). Although *endoxa* has become synonymous with *doxa*, the *appearance* of accuracy or truth is the distinction we emphasize since "*doxa* has a force that has nothing to do with Truth" (Amossy, 2002, p. 371).

The HBC pills' powerful, enduring *doxa* is rooted in the sexual revolution of the 1960s. Without a doubt, HBC has likely prevented conception in millions of situations and, when taken regularly, approximately 99% of the time. Importantly, current *doxa* on HBC suggests that HBC rescues women from unwanted pregnancies without physiological detriment. In so doing, these *doxas* distort and misrepresent the more complete picture of what HBC does to women's bodies, hormonally, through purposeful omission of information about possible risks.

Of course, we recognize HBC effectively prevents pregnancy through the various methods we describe next; however, *doxastic* beliefs about *how* these HBCs work chemically neither communicate nor contribute accurate knowledge about what happens hormonally and physiologically to women. In fact, the medical establishment's mismanagement of HBC knowledge has resulted in federal actions from the FDA and lawsuits against the pharmaceutical companies that manufacture HBCs—actions and cases we examine presently. Additionally, as corrective counterbalances to incomplete knowledge about HBC, we explain alternative discourses that honor the care and natural hormonal processes female bodies experience through ovulation and menses. Although HBC was once (and is currently) thought to be a benign, expedient choice that prevented pregnancy, once paired with alternative health discourses, a more complete picture of the hormonal work HBC prevents becomes evident. We see our scholarship as contributing to the ebb and flow of *doxa* and to efforts to upend *doxastic* beliefs about HBC by providing more complete knowledge about how HBC works.

Hormonal Birth Control

According to the Guttmacher Institute (2018), "Seventy-two percent of women who practice contraception currently use non-permanent methods, primarily hormonal methods (the pill, patch, implant, injectable and vaginal ring) …" (para. 13), which means 9.5 million women in the US have used the pill (Guttmacher Institute, 2018) or four out of five sexually experienced women (Daniels, Mosher, & Jones, 2013). Medical and pharmaceutical discourses prioritize effectiveness over health. Since very little of the science of hormones is explained to users, the discourses surrounding HBC reflect *doxa* that originates in profits-driven pharmaceutical marketing tactics and the acceptance of that control over women's bodies. The goal seems to be control at any cost, with no questions asked, rather than working to provide women with knowledge about what is happening in their bodies—information that might lead them to seek out alternative birth control methods.

For example, HBC effectively prevents conception by preventing ovulation. However, the cost of that kind of effectiveness is a disruption of women's hormonal and menstrual cycles. Since ovulation is the only way that women produce progesterone, HBC interrupts this process, which, according to the counter-discourses explored below, can have lasting negative impacts on women's bodies. HBC's curative function, i.e. inhibiting menses, ovulation, and progesterone production, effectively fulfills the motivation for studying women's sex hormones in the first place: controlling and sanitizing their bodies. HBC, then, does what it was originally intended to do—it "cures" women of their bodily functions, stripping down their hormonal response functions to render them less—in the discourse of the early twentieth century—female. However, the cost of preventing pregnancy with HBC—the loss of the natural progesterone-estrogen hormonal fluctuations—are virtually ignored by biomedically driven *doxa*.

It is common practice for OBGYNs to prescribe HBC not only to prevent pregnancy, but also to regulate periods and treat acne, severe menstrual cramps, endometriosis, fibroids, ovarian cysts, PCOS, and almost all female reproductive ailments. Although we do not want to diminish HBC's pain-relieving capacities, unfortunately, the impact of synthetic estrogen and progestins, and the ovulatory-prohibiting product of some forms of HBC, have been misrepresented and, in some cases, oversold to the public. And, like Briden (2014), we recognize birth control pills as "medicine for debilitating conditions such as severe endometriosis and very heavy periods" (para. 1). However, "What [we] don't celebrate is the distorted message that HBC is the only birth control. What [we] don't celebrate is its widespread prescription as 'hormone balance' for virtually any hormonal symptom that might arise in women and teenage girls" (para. 2).

Oral Contraceptives

In the last decade and a half, Bayer Healthcare Pharmaceuticals—the manufacturer of HBC pills Yasmin and Yaz released in 2001 and 2006, respectively—was named in 10,000 lawsuits for blood clots and death due to blood clots from these HBC pills (Grigg-Spall, 2012, paras. 2–3). Marketed to women in their twenties (Singer, 2009, para. 20), Yasmin and Yaz differ from other kinds of HBC pills because they contain a synthetic progesterone, drospirenone (Grigg-Spall, 2012, para. 1). Bayer promoted Yasmin and Yaz "as less likely to cause weight gain and bloating than other birth control pills" (Grigg-Spall, 2012, para. 1), which contravenes the FDA's guidelines regarding marketing drugs for any other reason than the FDA-approved uses (Singer, 2009, para. 14).

In 2008, Bayer aired two television ads set to popular music. According to Singer (2009), a Twisted Sister song, "We're not Gonna Take It," played in the background, while women "kicked away or punctured floating signs with labels like 'irritability' and 'feeling anxious'" (Singer, 2009, para. 21)—emotions often affiliated with menses. During the commercial, the narrator suggested that Yaz is "a pill that goes beyond the rest" and clears skin of blemishes (para. 21). Singer described a second video that made similar claims beyond preventing contraception, set to "Goodbye to You" by the Veronicas (Singer, 2009, para. 22).

In response to these ads, the Director of the Division of Drug Marketing, Advertising and Communications at the FDA, Thomas Abrams (2008), sent a letter stating that the Yaz ads were "misleading because they broaden the drug's indication, overstate the efficacy of YAZ, and minimize serious risks associated with the use of the drug" (Abrams, 2008, para. 1). However, "As part of an unusual crackdown on deceptive consumer drug advertising, the FDA and the attorneys general of 27 states required Bayer to run […] new ads to correct previous Yaz [2008] marketing," specifically mandating these advertisements state they do not cure either acne or PMS (Singer, 2009, para. 3).

Indeed, based upon its "aggressively screened commercials that were said to be making misleading assertions" about what the pill could do, including "unapproved uses and making light of the more serious health risks (such as blood clots)" (Grigg-Spall, 2012, para. 2), Bayer allocated $20 million at the behest of the FDA and the complaints of the state attorneys general. In fact, the revised $20 million advertising campaign was a result of Bayer walking back its statements of the benefits of these pills and the efforts of the FDA to hold Bayer accountable for distorting the pill's efficacy, intended uses, and "over-promis[ing] the benefits and minimiz[ing] the risks associated with YAZ" (Abrams, 2008, para. 1).

To meet the FDA's requirements to rectify the "deceptive consumer drug advertising" (Singer, 2009, para. 3), Bayer released a 2009 ad that reads:

> If you or your healthcare provider believes you have PMS, you should only take YAZ if you want to prevent pregnancy; and not for the treatment of PMS. Prescription YAZ is 99% effective at preventing pregnancy when taken as directed. YAZ may be used to treat moderate acne for women who are at least 14 years old, have started having menstrual periods and want to use the Pill for contraception.

Unfortunately for Bayer and consumers, the FDA also found issues with the ads for Yaz (and Mirena, the intrauterine contraceptive device, IUD) in 2009, citing Bayer "fail[ed] to communicate any risk information associated with the use of these drugs. In addition, the sponsored links for YAZ and Mirena inadequately communicate the drugs' indications, and the sponsored links for Mirena overstate the efficacy of the drug" (Doshi, 2009, para. 1). Additionally, "Bayer also [faced] lawsuits ... over its birth control pills, Yaz and Yasmin ... Bayer paid $750 million to settle Yaz lawsuits involving women who suffered blood clots, some fatal. Thousands of claims remain outstanding" (Llamas, 2013, para. 9).

IUDs

The Mirena website has a scrolling ad bar at the top, which rotates through three different images of women and children. The content of the images indicates that Mirena is a HBC method geared towards women aged 30 and over and for women who are already mothers. In each ad, a mother is happily holding her child; there is a light and carefree tone. The subheading for the ad reads "Birth control for busy moms," and one of the informational bullet points indicates "You don't have to take [it] every day." This form of birth control is meant to free up time in the hectic lives of mothers who may not be ready for more children. The ad bar states, "[it] can be removed at any time if you want to get pregnant," and, digging deeper into the literature about Mirena, the website indicates that the IUD is reversible and once removed women can try to get pregnant "right away" (Bayer, 2018a).

A section of the website titled "How Does Mirena Work to Prevent Pregnancy?" indicates that "Mirena works in several ways: however, it is not known exactly how these actions work together to prevent pregnancy" (Bayer, 2018a). The website continues to emphasize that once the IUD is removed, users can try to get pregnant right away; however, since it is clear that the developers and distributors don't know how Mirena actually prevents pregnancy, there may also be some confusion about how to get pregnant once Mirena is removed.

In fact, one of the possible side effects of removing the Mirena is a topic that numerous bloggers have discussed at length: the Mirena crash. Most of the women blogging about the Mirena crash claim that they discover what it is by searching for the symptoms they experience after Mirena has been removed. Most recently, a personal injury legal group in Florida has put together a number of legal cases against Bayer for the undisclosed side effects women experience after removal, including: runaway emotions, anxiety, and depression; mood swings that affect interpersonal relationships and professional performance; lethargy and fatigue; nausea, vomiting, and persistent stomach cramps; persistent breast tenderness; breakthrough bleeding; decreased sex drive and painful sex (Dolman Law Group, 2017, para. 1). According to almost 800 comments on the *Everything Mom* (2009) blog post "Mirena Crash," women also experience extremely heavy periods, clotting, and increased pain during their periods after Mirena is removed. The hormone imbalance that can be caused by the removal of the IUD and the hormones that control the thinning of the uterine lining and the thickening of cervical mucus can both contribute to the "crash" (Lockluff, 2015, para. 7).

Officially, Bayer does not acknowledge the Mirena crash, and the Q&A section of the Mirena website lists only the following as common side effects: placement disorder, expulsion, missed menstrual periods, changes in bleeding, cysts on the ovary (Bayer, 2018b). However, the complaints and complications extend beyond the Mirena crash. For example, "In July 2018, there were about 2,400 active Mirena lawsuits in New York and New Jersey. In April 2018, Bayer reported that it had reached a settlement in about 4,100 Mirena organ perforation lawsuits" (Llamas, 2018, para. 1). Additional lawsuits in these two states "blame Mirena for pressure buildup in the skull called pseudotumor cerebri or intracranial hypertension" (para. 3). Like Yaz, the failure to adequately communicate all of the potential risks associated with using Mirena seems to be a problem of increasing magnitude that has prompted former Mirena users and advocates to petition the FDA for a Mirena recall (para. 5). Thus, while advertisements for HBCs contribute to *doxastic* beliefs about the role of HBCs in women's reproductive health woes, women participating in grassroots efforts have forced pharmaceutical companies to take responsibility for the omitted nefarious side effects of HBCs and disrupted *doxa*. As we demonstrate below, CAM discourses also contribute to challenging existing *doxa* on HBC by offering women accurate information on the health benefits of their natural hormone cycles.

Naturopathic Medicine and CAM: What HBC Does, Hormonally

HBC falls directly into the nexus between legislative lobbying, fundraising efforts, and the advocacy efforts of non-biomedical practitioners who seek to intervene in decision-making about women's health in order to give women greater agency. Notable examples include Toni Weschler, MPH, and naturopath Lara Briden, who have intervened in this capacity by resisting mainstream medical knowledge that informs *doxa* and providing accurate information about reproduction, menses, and fertility. In the process, these corrective, alternative discourses provide opportunities for women to pursue reproductive freedom via other, natural methods, such as FAM, and to opt out of the pharmaceutical-industrial complex. Weschler and Briden provide opportunities for women to embrace and enjoy their hormonal and menstrual cycles and symptoms—another form of resistance to *doxa*. Their arguments and information function as counter-discourses, in so far as they call attention to information that is omitted from the mainstream, dominant, medical discourses. In so doing, they counteract the rhetorical force that is wielded by such omissions, providing other, natural methods that contribute to the same effect: preventing pregnancy.

Weschler's landmark text, *Taking Charge of Your Fertility* (*TCOYF*), was first published in 1995. A twentieth anniversary edition was released in 2015 (Weschler, 2015), along with an updated website, with resources and tools for the TCOYF method, which advocates the use of FAM to plan or prevent pregnancies. Usually understood by traditional medical practitioners as the rhythm method,[1] FAM is meant to serve as an educational tool to demystify women's complete hormonal cycle. It is important to note that this method is not as effective at preventing pregnancy as HBC. However, Weschler is explicit that in educating themselves about individual hormonal cycles, women have a better opportunity to get pregnant. She states that if preventing pregnancy is the purpose for using FAM, heterosexual couples must use a barrier method, or "double up on methods of birth control" (Weschler, 2015, p. 12), and that they must use protection constantly while getting familiar with the method in order to avoid pregnancy. Thus, women do not bear the burden of birth control alone. Weschler explicitly states: "FAM affords men the opportunity to lovingly and actively share in the responsibility of contraception" (p. 17).

Weschler's work was inspired by her experience in college. She was frustrated that a recurring medical problem was the "inevitable side effect of the various birth control methods [she] tried. If [she] wasn't dealing with weight gain and headache caused by the pill, [she] was enduring urinary tract infections from the diaphragm or irritation from the sponge" (Weschler, 2015, p. xix). Weschler initially wrote the book because she believes that:

> Your menstrual cycle is not something that should be shrouded in mystery. By the time you reach the end of this book, I hope you will also experience the liberation of feeling in control of your body. Beyond its practical value in giving you the tools to avoid or achieve pregnancy naturally and to take control of your gynecological health, this information about your cycle and body will empower you with numerous facets of self-knowledge that you rightly deserve.
>
> (*Weschler, 2015, p. xxi*)

Weschler assumes an audience that is interested in methods beyond HBC, and, as such, she spends very little time in the book discussing it. Instead, she focuses on bodily recovery once HBC is discontinued. Because FAM is individual and subjective, Weschler focuses on what counts as a normal cycle according to each person's individual patterns in their monthly cervical fluid, basal body temperature, and cervical position. She provides detailed charting tools, as well as charting examples throughout the book, with chapters geared toward avoiding pregnancy, getting pregnant, understanding conditions like PCOS and ovarian cysts, as well as the perimenopause and the menopause. Chapters such as "Troubleshooting Your Cycle: Expecting the Unexpected" demonstrate that Weschler's goal as a healthcare professional is to advocate for women's self-knowledge. *TCOYF* advocates charting and provides free resources in the form of blank charts, sample charts, and free iOS and Android apps.

The chart is meant to give women the ability, over the course of three months, to identify patterns in their monthly cycles so that they can discover what counts as their "normal." Weschler is clear that charting alone is not sufficient birth control, and that once women identify their fertile days, they should either abstain from sexual intercourse, or use an effective barrier method.

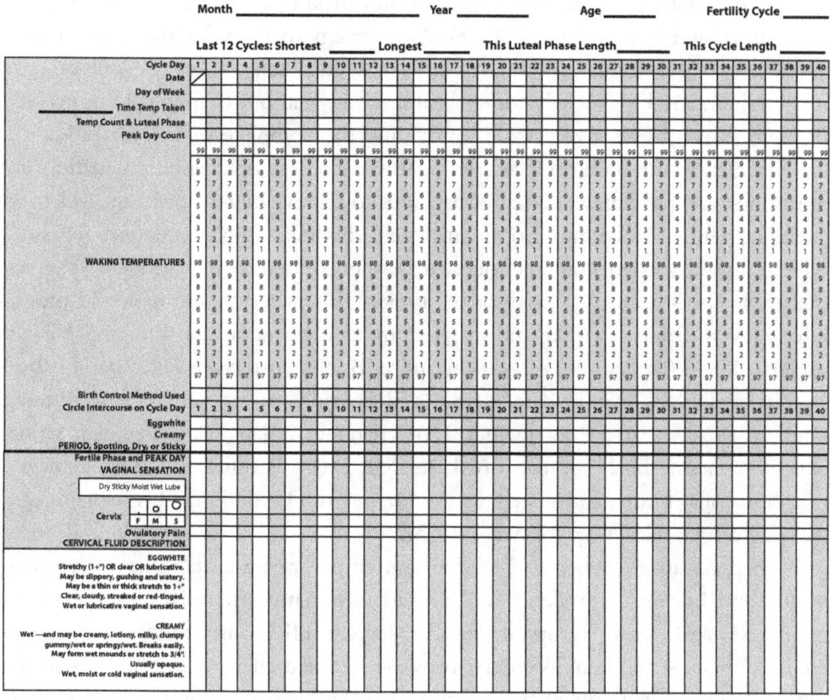

FIGURE 13.1 Weschler's template FAM chart
Source: Weschler, 2015

Relatedly, Briden's work as a naturopath led her to write *The Period Repair Manual* (Briden, 2017e), which has sold over 32,000 combined copies in two editions (L. Briden, personal communication, September 27, 2018). In tandem with her blog, Briden's (2018a) website announces her as "The Period Revolutionary" who:

> view[s] the body as a logical, regenerative system that knows what to do when it's given the right support. And in [her] twenty years of practice, [she's] seen that simple principle in action with thousands of patients. And [she's] learned that period problems respond incredibly well to nutrition and other natural treatments. *Period problems can be fixed without the band-aid solution of HBC.*
>
> *(emphasis added, para. 4)*

With over 175,000 (95,000 unique visitors) website visitors to larabriden.com in August 2018 and 5.74 million website views since 2012, as well as 17,600 Instagram and over 3,200 Twitter followers, using Twitter with the hashtag #ovulationmatters, Briden has called for medicine to do better. Briden's "mission is nothing short of fundamentally changing the way we view women's health. Namely, that ovulatory cycles are important for general health, not just making a baby" (L. Briden, personal communication, September 27, 2018). As a strategy to showcase the importance of ovulation in health, she has written blog posts addressing, "… every clinician, personal trainer, and blogger who offers health advice without thinking about periods" (Briden, 2018b). Her goals include providing the complete picture of HBCs and their ovulation-inhibiting effects, setting the record straight about ovulation and hormones, and providing alternative methods to achieve better menstrual cycles. For example, Briden advocates magnesium and rhodiola supplementation for stress, which can impact ovulation and menstrual cycles (Briden, 2017d; 2013b); Vitex and melatonin for hormonal sleep disorders typically impacted by estrogen and progesterone levels (Briden, 2013a); and magnesium, zinc, turmeric, and avoiding dairy for menstrual pain (Briden, 2017c). Furthermore, Briden corrects misinformation about conditions like PCOS (Briden, 2018c) and provides treatments for four different kinds of PCOS that do not include HBC (Briden, 2014). Like Weschler, Briden advocates natural birth control (FAM through Daysy Fertility Monitor), as well as non-hormonal birth control such as the copper IUD, condoms, Caya diaphragm, and Femcap Cervical Cap (Briden, 2017b).

Both practitioners work to broaden contemporary understanding of women's bodily and hormonal processes and provide alternatives to HBC for preventing pregnancy and, thus, disrupt *doxas* that suggest HBCs are clear, obvious, safe choices for most women. Weschler provides detailed charts and templates so that women can get to know their bodies and cycles, as well as how and why those cycles might change due to stress, aging, illness, lack of sleep, and pregnancy (to name just a few outlined issues). And Briden reconfigures the period, not as a messy bodily function to avoid, but as a hormonal cycle resulting in bleeding, identifying menstruation-related effects in order for females to understand their periods and symptoms. For example, HBC suppresses ovulation and menses, except, purportedly, in cases when there is a "pill bleed." A pill bleed is meant to simulate menses. However, according to Briden (2017a), "we don't need periods if a period is defined as a bleed. And we certainly don't need pill-bleeds which are nothing whatsoever to do with ovulation or beneficial hormones" (para. 10). However, she clarifies, "we do need periods if a period is defined as a hormonal cycle" (para. 11). Basically, it's the hormonal cycle that starts with ovulation, and without conception, ends with menses, that is overlooked and undervalued by existing *doxa* about HBC—a *doxa* reinforced by the ads analyzed in this chapter and a *doxa* Weschler and Briden counter.

Furthermore, in many cases the general public misunderstands the science behind hormonal contraception. It is erroneously thought that HBC contains estrogen and progesterone. More accurately, HBC contains synthetic versions of estrogen and progestins (Briden, 2015, para. 1). Briden (2015) clarified, "The progestins in HBC *are not progesterone*" (emphasis original). Additionally, Briden even pointed out that the *British Medical Journal* falsely conflated progesterone and progestins, stating: "They use the word progesterone when they really mean a progestin such as drospirenone, levonorgestrel, or medroxyprogesterone" (Briden, 2015, para. 2). The earliest birth control pills, specifically Enovid, contained a mix of norethynodrel (synthetic progesterone) and synthetic estrogen (Case Western Reserve University, n.d., para. 3). In fact, HBC usually contains "drugs ethinylestradiol, levonorgestrel, [medroxyprogesterone,] and drospirenone, which are the drugs of birth control and are not beneficial like our own hormones" (Briden, 2017a, para. 2).

Correcting *Doxa* as Activism by Accuracy

Weschler's and Briden's discourses show what is hidden in those cropped, *doxastic* pictures of biomedically presented HBCs. Based on the Yaz advertising complaints and Bayer corrective ads, the distortion of HBC persists and reinforces existing *doxa* surrounding HBC. Our argument hinges on the misconstrual of information about hormonal cycles, hormones, and HBC. The Yaz ads, whether the FDA-sanctioned ones from 2008 or the post-complaint, corrective advertisements from 2009, reinforce existing *doxa* surrounding HBC. As Weschler and Briden demonstrate, assumptions about the efficacy of HBC to prevent pregnancy, while merited, detract from the bigger picture about the importance of estrogen and progesterone, i.e., hormones and hormonal cycles that are integral to and indicators of women's reproductive health.

Our argument from the outset of this chapter has promoted the notion that HBC has fulfilled its original purpose—to control and sanitize women's bodies in pursuit of a social agenda that is cleansed of women's bodily functions, and the hormonal and menstrual cycles that produce them. For instance, Yaz advertised its HBC pill for purposes—ending PMS and treating acne—other than FDA-approved ones. As such, the ads for popular HBC tend to reinforce the *doxa* associated with hormones and women's bodies, i.e. they keep in check the bodily functions that are a part of normal hormonal and menstrual cycles.

Essentially, HBC *doxa* compromises women's health by underemphasizing and ignoring the importance of hormones and their cycles. By either knowing and withholding or not explaining "how these actions work together to prevent pregnancy," the ads demonstrate that knowledge about women's hormones and hormonal cycles is not prioritized. In fact, the priority of HBC is the same as it was in the early twentieth century: to cure women and control the hormones that make women physiologically women. In the process of sanitizing women's bodies, existing liberatory birth control *doxa* is simultaneously supported and reinforced. However, Weschler's and Briden's approaches privilege sharing the knowledge of HBC and women's hormonal and menstrual cycles. In these cases, the naturopathic discourses surrounding hormonal and menstrual cycles provide a counter-discourse—a corrective, active resistance to scientific and biomedical discourse and *doxa* about HBC.

The counter-discourse we identify does not obfuscate the liberatory possibilities of hormonal birth control, but it does provide a useful educational tool, and an alternative, for overcoming the truncated information provided by the medical industry to women about their reproductive cycles. Weschler's and Briden's work demonstrates the importance of hormonal and menstrual cycles for women's reproductive health and points to the significant work to be done in medical and scientific discourses surrounding understanding and informing women about their bodies' natural functions and cycles.

Our purpose in this chapter, in other words, is not to undo the positive work done for women by making HBC widely available. Indeed, access to birth control is a fundamental human right and must be defended, especially in the political climate of the US at present. Instead, we are interested in exploring the *doxastic* effects of HBC on women and their bodies and in exploring the only existing counter-discourse to dominant medical discourse around reproductive health. Our study demonstrates that the dominant medical discourse isolates women from basic knowledge about how their hormones function. The counter-discourse is available but demands work from women and possibly, discomfort. Charting and tracking cycles does not "cure" acne or cramps, but it does help women to understand how their bodies process their hormones throughout the course of their monthly cycles. Weschler's template does not prevent pregnancy on its own; but for women interested in reproductive health, it offers a distinctly embodied discourse that demands attention, detail, and, ultimately, a fully embodied experience. Such embodied rhetorical practices are ingenious as they have the capacity to disrupt recalcitrant forms of *doxa* that lead many women to uncritically embrace HBCs.

Note

1 A contraception method in which an individual tracks their menstrual history in an attempt to predict ovulation. Based on a 28-day cycle, 24 out of 100 women who use the rhythm method become pregnant in their first year (Mayo Clinic Staff, 2018, para. 7).

References

Abrams, T. (2008). "Warning letter." Retrieved from http://45ijagbx6du4a lbwj3e23cj1-wpengine.netdna-ssl.com/wp-content/uploads/2008-yaz-fda-warning.pdf
Altman, K.E. (1988). "Rhetorical and historical inquiry in the feminist reconstitution of knowledge." *Journal of Communication Inquiry*, 12(2), 24–38.
Amossy, R. (2002). "Introduction to the study of Doxa." *Poetics Today*, 23(3), 369–394.
Bayer Healthcare Pharmaceuticals. (2018a). "About Mirena. Effective birth control without a daily pill." Retrieved from www.mirena-us.com/about-mirena/
Bayer Healthcare Pharmaceuticals. (2018b). "Questions and answers about Mirena." Retrieved from www.mirena-us.com/q-and-a/
Bizzell, P. (2000). "Feminist methods of research in the history of rhetoric: What difference do they make?" *Rhetoric Society Quarterly*, 30(4), 5–17.
Briden, L. (n.d.). "About me." Retrieved from www.larabriden.com/about/
Briden, L. (2013a, December 9). "Help for hormonal sleep problems [blog post]." Retrieved from www.larabriden.com/what-to-do-about-hormonal-sleep-problems
Briden, L. (2013b, May 3). "How Rhodiola shelters us from stress and cortisol [blog post]." Retrieved from www.larabriden.com/how-rhodiola-shelters-us-from-stress-and-cortisol/
Briden, L. (2014, May 16). "Treatment for 4 types of PCOS. Treat the cause [blog post]." Retrieved from www.larabriden.com/treatment-for-4-types-of-pcos-treat-the-cause
Briden, L. (2015, October 6). "The crucial difference between progesterone and progestins [blog post]." Retrieved from www.larabriden.com/the-crucial-difference-between-progesterone-and-progestins/
Briden, L. (2017a, September 30). "Do women need periods? [blog post]." Retrieved from www.larabriden.com/do-women-need-periods/
Briden, L. (2017b, August 23). "The 5 best types of natural birth control [blog post]." Retrieved from www.larabriden.com/quick-survey-5-best-types-of-natural-birth-control
Briden, L. (2017c, February 11). "When period pain is not normal [blog post]." Retrieved from www.larabriden.com/when-period-pain-is-not-normal
Briden, L. (2017d, March 6). "Why stress hits hard in your 40s [blog post]." Retrieved from www.larabriden.com/real-reason-stress-hits-hard-in-your-40s-adrenal
Briden, L. (2017e). *Period repair manual*. (2nd ed.). London: Pan Macmillan.
Briden, L. (2018a). "Lara Briden, the period revolutionary." Retrieved from wws.larabriden.com
Briden, L. (2018b, April 3). "If you're not thinking about ovulation, you're not thinking about health [blog post]." Retrieved from www.larabriden.com/ovulation-is-a-sign-of-health/
Briden, L. (2018c, September 3). "Maybe it's not PCOS [blog post]." Retrieved from www.larabriden.com/you-might-not-have-pcos
Case Western Reserve University. (n.d.). "History of contraception: Oral contraceptive pill." Retrieved from https://case.edu/affil/skuyhistcontraception/online-2012/pill.html
Crowley, S. (2006). *Toward a civil discourse: Rhetoric and fundamentalism*. Pittsburgh, PA: University of Pittsburgh Press.

Daniels, K., Mosher, W.D., & Jones, J. (2013). "Contraceptive methods women have ever used: United States, 1982–2010." *National Health Statistics Reports*, 62, 1–15. Retrieved from www.cdc.gov/nchs/data/nhsr/nhsr062.pdf.

Dolman Law Group (2017). "The Mirena crash is real and it's affecting countless women." Retrieved from www.dolmanlaw.com/mirena-crash-lawyers/

Doshi, S. (2009). "Corrective action letter." Retrieved from http://45ijagbx6du4a lbwj3e23cj1-wpengine.netdna-ssl.com/wp-content/uploads/2009-yaz-fda-warning.pdf

Everything Mom. (2009). "Mirena crash: The Mirena IUD side effects after removal." Retrieved from www.everythingmom.com/health/mirena-crash-the-mirena-iud-si de-effects-after-removal

Frank, R.T. (1929). *The female sex hormone.* Springfield, IL: Charles T. Thomas.

Gibbons, M.G. (2014). "Beliefs about the mind as doxastic inventional resource: Freud, neuroscience, and the case of Dr. Spock's baby and child care." *Rhetoric Society Quarterly*, 44(5), 427–448.

Grigg-Spall, H. (2012, February 9). "Just how safe is Yaz? Women need to know! [blog post]." Retrieved from http://msmagazine.com/blog/2012/02/09/just-how-safe-is-ya z-women-need-to-know/

Guttmacher Institute. (2018). "Contraceptive use in the United States." Retrieved from www.guttmacher.org/fact-sheet/contraceptive-use-united-states

Koerber, A. (2018). *From hysteria to hormones: A rhetorical history.* University Park, PA: Pennsylvania State University Press.

Llamas, M. (2013). "FDA approves Skyla, first new IUD since Mirena arrived in 2000." Retrieved from www.drugwatch.com/news/2013/01/18/fda-approves-skyla-first-new-iud-since-mirena-arrived-in-2000/

Llamas, M. (2018). "Mirena lawsuits." Retrieved from www.drugwatch.com/mirena/la wsuits/

Lockluff, M. (2015). "So this is the dreaded Mirena crash (and burn)." Retrieved from http s://adventuresofmel.com/so-this-is-the-dreaded-mirena-crash-and-burn

Mayo Clinic Staff. (2018). "Rhythm method for natural family planning." Retrieved from www.mayoclinic.org/tests-procedures/rhythm-method/about/pac-20390918

Royster, J.J. & Kirsch, G. (2012). *Feminist rhetorical practices: New horizons for rhetoric, composition, and literacy studies.* Carbondale, IL: Southern Illinois University Press.

Singer, N. (2009). "A birth control pill that promised too much." *The New York Times.* Retrieved from www.nytimes.com/2009/02/11/business/worldbusiness/11iht-11pill. 20100508.html

Weschler, T. (2015). *Taking charge of your fertility: The definitive guide to natural birth control, pregnancy achievement, and reproductive health, 20th anniversary edition.* New York: Harper-Collins Publishers.

Woods, C. (2012). "(Im)mobile metaphors: Toward an intersectional rhetorical history." In K. Chávez and C. Griffin (Eds.). *Standing in the intersection: Feminist voices, feminist practices in communication studies* (pp. 78–96). Albany, NY: SUNY Press.

14

ALTERING IMAGINARIES AND DEMANDING TREATMENT

Women's AIDS Activism in Toronto, 1980s–1990s

Janna Klostermann

Taking a queer, feminist approach to rhetorical inquiry, this chapter examines women's AIDS activism in Toronto in the late 1980s and early 1990s through the archival materials available through the AIDS Activist History Project (AAHP) and the Canadian Lesbian and Gay Archives. I trace the historically situated, ordinary, and collective work that women AIDS activists did to revise their lives and to transform social relations and imaginaries—or the assumed picture of "who" gets AIDS in the minds of the government, citizens, and other AIDS activists. Drawing on activist interviews and archival materials, I contribute to collective projects of remembering for the future by attending to the dramatically underdocumented history of (women's) AIDS activism in Canada (Kinsman, 2018; Shotwell, 2016a). Building on Scott's (2003) foundational work on HIV testing and the rhetorics that create and sustain ideas of who is at risk of contracting HIV, I ask: What rhetorical and material work did women AIDS activists and women living with HIV/AIDS do? To what extent did their work involve—symbolically and materially—(re)shaping their lives, social relations, and imaginaries? I review rhetorical studies, introduce the queer methods of scavenging and storying, and then clarify how activists worked to: 1) alter imaginaries of AIDS through protests and publications; and 2) alter treatment relations through pamphlets and support groups.

This chapter extends studies in rhetoric by attending to, making public, and theorizing the rhetorical and material work involved in altering social relations and imaginaries. Social imaginaries are "social in the broadest sense" as they sustain the "received politics of knowledge" (Code, 2006, pp. 30, 194), and hold invitations and meanings about how relationships and responsibilities are configured (Armstrong, & Braedley, 2013). Informed by the research and thinking of feminist sociologist Smith (2005), I apply an expanded definition of "work" to account for "anything done by people that takes time and effort, that they mean to do, that is done under definite conditions" (pp. 151–152). I attend to activists' ordinary and often underacknowledged work, making visible "the utterly mundane and everyday situated accomplishment of largely taken-for-granted social situations" (de Montigny, 2017, p. 334). Taken together, these perspectives allow me to make visible AIDS activists' everyday collective work to shift relations of power and inequality and to open up new possibilities for women living with AIDS.

Tracing Symbolic and Material Effects of Women's Health Activism

> While Sue herself had put an initial, early stop to my disciplinary self-doubt ("Who gives a shit about rhetoric [...]?"), when her abdomen swelled painfully, we sat together in despair and words failed me.
>
> *(Restaino, 2015, p. 86)*

Writing with and in memoriam to her friend Susan Lundy Maute, Restaino (2015) grapples with how feminist rhetorical work might begin with our own lived experiences and struggles. Other feminist scholars commit similarly to using scholarly tools to understand human, embodied, material experiences and struggles (Klostermann, 2018; Smith, 2005; Stenberg, 2018). With a feminist orientation, I seek to conduct research from women's material standpoints, to attend to their real work, and to explicate their participation in (and in opposition to) lived social relations. Rhetorical approaches provide a guide for exploring women's health activism, directing our attention to the symbolic—to circulating terms and discourses—as well as to material conditions that shape rhetorical practices and possibilities.

Rhetoricians have long underscored the importance of attending to terms and the values backing them. As Emmons (2009) puts it, "words matter." Recent studies examine how health discourses circulate publicly across time and space, opening up fissures for social change (Agnew, 2018; Loyd, 2014). Taking a rhetorical approach centrally involves examining people's capacity to use language—or rhetorical forms, in particular—to shift power structures and public consciousness, while shifting cultural values, norms and preoccupations (Agnew, 2018, p. 271; Dubriwny, 2012; Hensley Owens, 2015). Some rhetoricians track shifting cultural perspectives of health discourses, while others explore how people rhetorically, creatively, and authorially respond to the circumstances of their health (see, for instance, Segal, 2012; and Hensley Owens, this collection).

Rhetorical analysis uncovers terms and narratives that deeply shape people's experiences (Garland-Thomson, 2007, 2015; Segal, 2015; Tadros, this collection); conventional, internalized "rules for speaking" (Segal, 2012); or messages about how to be ill (e.g., become "positive, courageous and combative" about cancer, rather than "weak, tired, discouraged" [Segal, 2012, p. 312]).[1] As Selzer (1999) put it, "rhetoric has long been concerned with the situatedness of literate acts and the real effects of discourse rather than with ideal possibilities" (p. 9). Focusing on the art of persuasion, Segal (2015) writes that "the rhetorical analyst's central question is 'who is persuading whom or what, and what are the means of persuasion?'" (p. 915). Attending to symbolic aspects, other questions to ask include: How do health discourses circulate publicly across time and space, promoting social change (Agnew, 2018; Loyd, 2014)? What are the terms and values backing them? What are shifting portrayals and valuations of a set phenomenon (e.g., of care, of an illness, or of people with an illness)? What incidents does the representation narrate (Garland-Thomson, 2015)?

Studies of rhetoric also attend to the relationship between materiality and rhetorical production (Agnew, 2018, p. 272; Burke, 1984; George, & Selzer, 2007, p. 110; Selzer, 1999, p. 9). Underscoring that meanings have social and material aspects, and that terms begin in action rather than knowledge (Burke, 1984, p. 274), rhetoricians clarify how our rhetorical practices and possibilities are shaped by our embodied presences and our social and material conditions (Agnew, 2018; Garland-Thomson, 2007; Selzer, 1999). They also note that our metaphors have material consequences (Agnew, 2018). For example, contributing to feminist studies of rhetoric as well as feminist critical disability studies, Garland-Thomson (2007) emphasizes "Our shapes, in all their uncontained variation, structure our stories" (p. 121). As she puts it, "shape or body is crucial, not incidental, to story; it makes story visible; in a sense it is story" (pp. 113–114). In her study of cancer rhetorics, Agnew (2018) also attends to the "embodied experiences of patients" and to the "material conditions that ground all communicative acts" (p. 292). She underscores that discourses are grounded in local practices and relations—in "material reality constituted by embodied encounters" (p. 275).

Queer Feminist Orientation: Scavenging and Storying

> Re-vision—the act of looking back, of seeing with fresh eyes, of entering an old text from a new critical direction—is for women more than a chapter in cultural history: it is an act of survival.
>
> *(Rich, 1972, p. 18)*

In addition to concern for the symbolic and material, this chapter takes a queer, feminist approach to rhetorical inquiry. It began with my work with the AAHP, a project, spearheaded by Alexis Shotwell and Gary Kinsman, that explores the social histories of AIDS activists the late 1980s and mid-1990s in Canada. Following Alexander and Wallace (2009), who underscore the "critical power of queerness" (p. 301), and following Waite (2015), who clears spaces for queer feminist approaches in composition research and pedagogy, I do the queer work of "combin[ing] methods that are often cast as being at odds with each other" (Halberstam, as cited by Waite, 2015, p. 59). I employ theorized methods of scavenging and story making (Rice, & Mündell, 2018; Waite, 2015).

Taking a queer approach comes with the invitation to disrupt normative practices, processes, and ways of knowing (Waite, 2015), rather than engaging in linear, responsible, straightforward work. Further, taking a feminist approach comes with the invitation to start with women's relations and struggles (Baines, & Daly, 2015; Smith, 2005), tracing their realization in and in relation to extended social relations and discourses. The goal is to interrogate social relations of struggle, while also contributing to collective projects of transforming them. I consider activists as expert practitioners of their lives (Smith, 2005), articulating their experiences and struggles (in conversation with Kinsman and Shotwell), and shedding light on the social relations of which they are a part. Aiming for revolution, not reform (Lorde, as cited by Waite, 2015, p. 67), I engaged in rhetorical inquiry—scavenging, storying, and seeking to clarify how life is symbolically and materially (re)produced through ordinary and collective rhetorical work.

My research involved scavenging through archival materials and activist interviews. Scavenging involves deep listening, perverse reading (Sedgwick, 2006), and the ordinary work of collecting scraps, fragments, or lesser-attended to, not-always-productive pieces (Waite, 2015). Waite (2015) writes that scavengers draw from "surprising places to disrupt [themselves] and their usual ways of 'knowing'" (p. 61). Scavenging is a way of "refusing coherence" by instead combining or bringing together the "seemingly unrelated" (Waite, 2015, p. 54). I scavenged oral history interviews with Toronto-based activists, along with other primary source materials, including posters, pamphlets, photographs, and news clippings. In scavenging, my aim was to "bring in alternative knowledge" (Stenberg, 2006, p. 146), while turning toward and revealing social contractions or tensions (Waite, 2015). I also tried to attend to the ordinary work people did—the queer moves they made—regardless of whether or not that work was "productive."

Storying—a dialectical, reflexive mode of relating—was also central to my work. Following recent invitations to blend artistic representations with scholarly writing (Ellingson, 2015), I experimented with engaging a different mode of feminist writing to tell a story about the ordinary and collective work of women AIDS activists. Rather than taking a "god's-eye view," and rather than seeking to produce a standard academic account that employs conceptual, professional, objectifying discourse (de Montigny, 2017), I sought to represent activists' situated, relational work, experiences, and knowledge. I narrowed in on the stories and memories of Darien Taylor, an AIDS activist and woman living with AIDS, who reflected on her work and on the social tensions involved in that work in her 2014 AAHP interview with Kinsman and Shotwell. I committed myself to storying and to taking people's stories seriously.

My research traces the cultural and historical shift from the "gay plague" to the lived sense that "women get AIDS, too." Taylor's stories offer evidence of the historically specific and collective work that AIDS activists/patients did to survive. Her interview, along with archival materials, brings into view some of the ways that AIDS activists revised their lives, while also reorganizing and reimagining relations and discourses about AIDS. In the remainder of the chapter, I explain the rhetorical/material context and historical conditions of the time, including the government inaction that activists were up against. From there, I focus on two rhetorical interventions made by activists to: 1) alter imaginaries of AIDS by representing and talking about women; and 2) alter treatment relations by supporting women with testing and treatment issues. I close by attending to the queer, rhetorical work (whether or not it was productive) involved in shifting social relations and imaginaries.

Stopping the Dying and Addressing the Fear: On the Rhetorical/ Material Conditions

Many of the AIDS activists interviewed by the AAHP described coming together to care for people who were getting sick and dying of AIDS, as the government, or public health in particular, was doing nothing (Barnett, 2014; Brown, 2014; Kinsman, 2014; McCaskell, 2014). Writing in *Rites* magazine at the time, activist ethnographer George W. Smith (n.d.) recalled a man with AIDS and dementia being attacked by police: "tear gas[sed], … captured, strapped into a stretcher and taken to the Toronto General" ("Talking politics: Police shape politics of AIDS"). Elaborating on these conditions, Taylor (2014) shed light on her own difficulties accessing treatment in the mid-1980s as a woman living with HIV. She said:

> … I was just so frightened and ashamed. Not knowing where to start, and it was hard to find where to start. Well, you know, there was no Internet first of all. So, it was like, a telephone book. You look up AIDS or HIV and there's nothing there. So, I started by going to my family doctor, who wasn't my doctor, it was my parents' doctor, and he was completely … I guess, frightened, but uninformed. And the information that he gave me was really just, basically, his biases. But he did give the name of the doctor that was treating people with HIV. Then I, through that, managed to piece the little path together … I remember going to see the AIDS doctor in Hamilton—Stephan Landis. He was giving me information, and at one point he made a mistake and he said, "… and when you shave …" He was talking to me about razors because he'd just been telling men about shaving. It was like, "I shave my legs, is that what you're talking about?" [laughter] He was just so used to giving that information to gay men that he, in some way, hadn't quite taken … I don't know exactly what it is, but that kind of mistake was something that happened quite often. In the beginning it wasn't quite in their vocabulary yet to distinguish between men and women with HIV.

> *(Taylor, 2014, pp. 4–5)*

Taylor powerfully narrated the lack of services and the ways the medical establishment had been directing their attention and care to men.

Similarly, Toronto activist Renee du Plessis (2014) described the emotionally challenging conditions in the hospitals as "disturbing," as she witnessed "over-the-top-reactionary" healthcare workers "dressing up in their masks and responding to [a person living with AIDS] not as a person but as a contamination" (p. 3) As she put it, healthcare workers would "refuse to touch the chart of somebody who was designated as having AIDS" (p. 3).

In their AAHP interviews, many activists highlighted the government inaction at the time, calling attention to harmful, limited or non-existent supports, practices, and policies centered on harassing, quarantining, and criminalizing HIV/AIDS positive people (Conrad, & Shotwell, 2018). Shotwell (2016b) writes: "The conditions for life with HIV and AIDS were both biochemical (was there medicine that could treat the syndrome) and social (was there a place to live, food, people who would touch you)" (p. 3). She points to the "policy, institutional, practical, and medical conditions that would make it possible to live" (p. 5).

Speaking back to these conditions, and to the devaluation and degradation of people living with AIDS, activists working in Toronto wanted both to "stop, or slow down at least, the dying that [was] taking place" (McCaskell, 2014, p. 4), and to "address in some small way the ignorance and fear that was around" (du Plessis, 2014, p. 1). One way was in organizing: many came together in the late 1980s to found AAN!, an action-oriented, committee-based group where Toronto-based activists mobilized a political strategy and worked *collectively* to transform the social organization of AIDS treatment. AAN! became well known for transforming AIDS treatment by supporting public funding for education, prevention, and treatment and service access (Barnett, 2014). AAN! is also well known for protesting against inhumane practices (such as clinical trials, quarantine camps), advocating for the release of drugs, reworking the Emergency Drug Release Program (a program centered on releasing drugs on compassionate grounds), and introducing Ontario's Trillium Drug Program (a program that continues to operate today) (Shotwell, 2016b). The group worked to understand the government apparatus and health institutions, and to learn about AIDS as an embodied, biomedical condition (Conrad, & Shotwell, 2018; Shotwell, 2016b). They contributed to shifting from seeing people as "AIDS victims" to people living with AIDS—recognizing/remaking AIDS as a "chronic manageable condition" (Conrad, & Shotwell, 2018). They engaged in radical rhetorical and material work to shift social imaginaries and relations of AIDS, which I elaborate on below by analyzing two particular interventions.

Voices of Women: Altering Social Imaginaries of AIDS

Scavenging this social history, I was struck by the rhetorical work of women AIDS activists to write women into the movement by leveraging the voices of women and speaking to women in particular. For instance, Taylor (2014) remembered taking to the streets—carrying a "women's banner in one of the Pride marches" (p. 30), and sporting a t-shirt to an International Women's Day event that read: "Women get AIDS. Get active" (p. 29). Another intervention that stands out is Taylor's work with Andrea Rudd to produce an anthology, *Positive Women: Voices of Women Living with AIDS*. The anthology responds to the "rhetorical needs" of the cultural moment—needs that are "fillable 1) only in writing, 2) for a specific audience, and 3) for the purpose of engaging that audience rhetorically (to act)" (Siegel Finer, 2016, p. 177). Elaborating on the need for the anthology, Taylor (2014) recalled it was written at a time when there "were no AIDS organizations for women" and when "we didn't know a single other HIV-positive woman in any other place in the world" (p. 19). It was also written at a time when men were saying, "What the fuck is she talking about women and HIV for? This is about gay men" (as one AIDS activist put it in his AAHP interview). The imaginaries at work in regard to AIDS offered a picture of a single type of patient: men.

Taylor (2014) outlined the work involved in producing the anthology—elaborating on their behind-the-scenes work to secure funding, to send out calls for submissions to women's organizations across the world, and to translate it into eight different languages. At a time when AIDS was being framed as a gay men's health issue, a key contribution that women made to the AIDS movement was "naming the fact that women do get HIV and there are all kinds of women who get it" (Barnett, 2014, p. 23). They worked to figure women into the movement, to "get women's issues front and centre," and to help others acknowledge that "women get AIDS too" (Barnett, 2014, p. 20). They gave "a face and a name to a lot of the issues that women were facing when testing positive or even being put on the agenda to get tested" (Barnett, 2014, p. 23)—writing themselves in and making themselves visible. Through their rhetorical work with the anthology, Taylor and Rudd presented a global AIDS analysis, put women's voices in conversation, and contributed to shifting public understanding of AIDS from a "gay disease" to something that shapes their lives and many other lives, too. They brought visibility to women's issues and inspired public recognition of women with AIDS, but also advocated awareness of AIDS as a public health issue that everyone should take seriously. They said, along with others, "Wait a minute, it's not just about gay men. There are also increasing infection rates among women" (Sri, 2014, p. 13).

The anthology and other interventions like it were also generative in that they revealed social tensions within the movement. So, while the anthology responded to real rhetorical needs, and worked for particular changes, it also revealed, or helped to illuminate, social tensions between rhetorical interventions centered on people's voices (often referred to as "representation" today) and practical, medical interventions around life-or-death needs—interventions perhaps seen as more of a priority. Chambers (2001) writes:

Writing criticism in the midst of an epidemic can feel uncomfortably like getting on with one's needlework while the house burns down. One ought to be dialing 911, rousing sleeping children and ushering them to safety, rescuing the cat or the strongbox that holds the insurance policy and the title deed. One ought to be working with ACT-UP, hassling congress people, contributing to AIDS research. What, Eric Michaels wondered in 1988, after reading the special AIDS issue of *October,* can criticism do? Can it fight disease, save lives?

(p. vii)

Following Chambers, some Toronto-based activists found it hard to justify devoting time or energy to issues of "voice" in the face of people's life-or-death need for medical treatment. For example, Toronto activist Brent Southin (2014) remembered thinking, "'Hey, these people are going to be dead,' and most of them within eighteen months, at that point, was the norm" (p. 22).

Like Southin, other activists talked about having to prioritize treatments, as opposed to attending to other social issues, and, pointedly, women-specific issues. The focus was on getting treatments into (men's) bodies. Yet, Chambers (2001) explains that "rhetoric *also* plays a not insignificant part" (p. vii), and that "when it is not possible to fight disease, save lives, or escape pain, it is still important to bear witness to that impossibility" (p. vii). So, while some activists couldn't remember any concrete women-specific proposals or political actions that everybody got behind, they talked about the importance of making visible women's lives or putting women's faces and names to it (Barnett, 2014; Taylor, 2014). As Taylor (2014) put it, "I think it was more about visibility for the issue than it was about specific concrete proposals" (p. 30). Through their rhetorical interventions, women made space for themselves and heightened the profile of their voices. Revealing and dwelling in this tension—between the symbolic and the material—was part of how the movement expanded possibilities for living otherwise—i.e., as people living with AIDS who did not fit the popular imagination.

Living Longer: Testing and Treating Women as a Way to Alter Relations of Care

The task was prevention. I guess in their mind they thought what I wanted was information about how not to transmit the virus, which was not the least bit interesting to me because I wasn't having sex. I could scarcely conceive of a time when I was ever going to want to have sex. I wanted to know what to do to live longer. That was radical then. That was not thought about and there were no answers, really.

(Taylor, 2014, p. 9)

Taylor's quote above offers a connection between the symbolic and the material in regard to women's rhetorical interventions on the scene of AIDS activism in

Toronto in the 1980s and 1990s. While doctors were focused on prevention for HIV-negative people, Taylor, herself an HIV-positive person, needed treatment. Her experience speaks to the extremity of effects that the lack of representation of women had during the AIDS crisis. It also provides an example of the necessity of the symbolic in effecting change for the better in the material.

To this cause, women AIDS activists worked to provide treatment support to women in particular. Speaking back to the government's focus on prevention, women both identified and called attention to gaps in the way women were being mistreated or refused testing, while also working to shift these practices. Taylor (2014) reflected on a few initiatives that she was involved in,[2] including a controversial pamphlet on women and AIDS that she produced with Mary Louise and Helen Humphries in 1990 or 1991 (p. 11).

When it comes to "rhetorical needs" (Siegel Finer, 2016), the pamphlet was an important intervention into the treatment landscape, as it was produced at a time when women were trying to understand their bodies in terms of "unknowable medical, physical things" (Shotwell, in Taylor, 2014, p. 21), when the government was directing its energy to prevention materials for HIV-negative people, and when limited treatment materials were addressing gay men (Taylor, 2014). It came at a time when women's bodies were being misread, mistreated, or refused testing (Taylor, 2014). It came at a time when "prevention pamphlets looked expensive and glossy and sexy and fun," while "treatment brochures … were kind of a granola paper, a bit newsprinty" (Taylor, 2014, p. 19). As Taylor (2014) put it, "You could really see the values" (p. 19) in the material construction of prevention/men/HIV-negative messages and treatment/women/HIV-positive messages.

The pamphlet helped to shift relations of care by acknowledging the fact of women living with AIDS and addressing them as the audience. The pamphlet read: "In the popular imagination, AIDS attacks only white, gay men. Yet in Canada, as in the rest of the world, ♀♀ *[women] are the fastest growing group of HIV/ARC/AIDS sufferers*" ("WOMEN GET A.I.D.S.," n.d.). Taylor further recalled the effect the pamphlet had on the audience, offering authoritative medical information to the best of their ability: "what we did was created substitutes for people's doctors. If you got these symptoms then you've got this disease, and you need this drug, and make sure that you ask your doctor about it. Because they don't necessarily know and people didn't know, and we spent a lot" (p. 17). The pamphlet also filled in an important gap by responding to issues around women's treatment, engaging with a "new language that was being created" (p. 22), engaging in an "examination of treatments that was really, really minute" (p. 28), and asking questions about whether "these treatments, which are tested mostly, exclusively in men, [are] appropriate for women" (p. 28).

Taylor described responding to issues around clinical trials, around women-specific infections being included in the definition of AIDS (p. 28), and around identifying various treatments for women (including around candidiasis, reproductive impacts, frequency of pap smears). Part of what they were working out were questions about what to do with/as women living with AIDS—how to articulate, advocate, and clear space.

While the pamphlet contributed to expanding possibilities, it also revealed social tensions and involved some disappointments with its reception. This is important to note, because although rhetorical interventions "stage moments when it could become otherwise," they "are not equal to changing the world" (Berlant, 2006, p. 35). One of the problems with focusing on treatment issues was that activists came up against a wall of language that was "way beyond what anyone even with education in university" was able to grasp (Southin, 2014, p. 31). Focusing on access to trials and treatment involved a lot of "insider knowledge," with complicated issues and with a "specialized vocabulary around treatment" (Mykhalovskiy, 2014, p. 5). Activists' ability to engage with "government and Pharma and researchers" (McCaskell, 2014, p. 31) and "to articulate what the politic would be" (Barnett, 2014, p. 4) was shaped by social differences related to class, race, gender, and education (Barnett, 2014; du Plessis, 2014; McCaskell, 2014), as well as to how "socially, politically, and financially informed" people were (Barnett, 2014, p. 4). This made for a limiting message and reach to the audience of women who needed more than a pamphlet.

Working from a queer perspective calls our attention to these unproductive or limited aspects of people's work. Attending to this work tells us not only about activists' lives and commitments, but about the rhetorical and material structures that they worked in relation to. In the case of people living with AIDS in Toronto in the 1980s and 1990s, they were up against forces so much larger in nature, number, and resources that they were often overwhelmed and angered by them. In her AAHP interview, Barnett (2014) asserted that AIDS was symbolic of a "complete and utter capitalist crisis, that's not of the market alone. It's the result—it's the capitalist crises of humanity. AIDS is symbolic to me of that. It's gender, race, class, sexuality, desire, and economics intertwined" (p. 32). Her thinking here sheds light on the enormous (normative, oppressive, deadly) social or institutional forces (government, market forces, medical industry, etc.) shaping people's everyday lives and inviting rhetorical arguments and actions counter to the establishment's cause.

While much of the work AIDS activists did was generative, as they "seize[d] on the unique opportunity of a fleeting moment to create new rhetorical possibility" (Miller, & Shepherd, 2004, para. 5), Taylor reflects on pulling back or drifting away from the movement, and she second-guesses the effectiveness of some of her rhetorical efforts. It's important to note that space doesn't always open up or that projects centered on "self-revising and relational reconfiguring" (Rice, & Mündell, 2018, p. 229) don't always work. Life-building projects don't always work, and people don't always become different in a way they can build a world on (Berlant, 2006, p. 26). Rhetorical interventions are "queer" in that the work they do or seek to accomplish is not always productive, straightforward or responsible. They can be both fruitful, lasting, and ingenious—and unproductive, fleeting, and futile. Rhetorical interventions are interesting in that they reveal possibilities and limits. They reveal the social in new ways—igniting new ways of seeing and disrupting normative relations and discourses.

Conclusion

In exploring the work of women AIDS activists who contributed to transforming understanding of AIDs and relations of care in Canada in the 1980s and 1990s, I traced the queer moves they made to symbolically and relationally constitute themselves, while shifting imaginaries and social relations. Speaking back to "gay plague" rhetoric, the movement involved embodied performances and public claims that "women get AIDS too" (that in some ways cut across bodies and across "pretty narrow, pretty limited" silences). Collectively, the movement worked for concrete material changes to treatment relations—getting medication into people's bodies; expanding access to treatment, trials, and drug-funding; providing women-specific information and supports.

By tracing the possibilities and tensions at the heart of this work, I have tried to show the utility of engaging in rhetorical inquiries that begin in people's everyday lives and examine their daily/nightly relations and struggles. Starting in people's everyday lives and attending to the individual and collective work they do provides a fitting way to ground rhetorical work. It also provides a situated way to explore the practical work involved in revising ways of living, relating, or imagining. So, remembering for the future (Shotwell, 2016a), and grasping that some lives are "nourished and others are shut down" (Shotwell, 2013, p. 114), I advocate "non-normative, contradictory, and strange" moves (Waite, 2015) and concrete material changes that work against the systemic inequities and normative relations that shape the lives of people with intensifying struggles or intensifying experiences of discrimination, heteronormativity, or state-based violence. Having revisited the ways women AIDS activists fought to broaden the focus from being a "Canadian Gay Men's Health Crisis" (Sri, 2014, p. 22) to testing, treating, and talking about women, I stand with Taylor, who, at the time of the 2014 interview, was concerned about the AIDS Committee of Toronto becoming a "gay men's health organization" (p. 31), and concerned about the way "prevention [has] re-entered the way we think about AIDS" (p. 31). I stand with Taylor and with others working out how to reimagine, reorganize, and expand possibilities for living *otherwise*.

Notes

1 Segal (2015) writes, "We all experience distress in the terms available for us to experience it in" (p. 916). Similarly, Garland-Thomson (2007) notes that narratives "frame our understandings of raw, unorganized experience" (p. 122).
2 Taylor (2014) recalled contributing to *AIDS ACTION NEWS!* and producing an article for *Healthsharing* (a major feminist publication in Canada focused on women's

health). Taylor's was the first article in the Canadian context written from the stand-point of a woman who was HIV-positive (p. 9). Importantly, Taylor distinguished between "prevention and treatment," while elaborating on "what a woman who finds out she's HIV-positive might want to do with her life" (p. 9).

References

Agnew, L. (2018). "Ecologies of cancer rhetoric: The shifting terrain of us cancer wars, 1920–1980." *College English*, 80(3), 271–296.

Alexander, J., & Wallace, D. (2009). "The queer turn in composition studies: Reviewing and assessing an emerging scholarship." *College Composition and Communication*, 61(1). W300–W320.

Armstrong, P., & Braedley, S. (Eds.) (2013). *Troubling care: Critical perspectives on research and practices.* Toronto, ON: Canadian Scholars' Press.

Baines, D., & Daly, T. (2015). "Resisting regulatory rigidities: Lessons from front-line care work." *Studies in Political Economy*, 95(1), 137–160.

Barnett, J. (2014). "Interview by Alexis Shotwell and Gary Kinsman." *AIDS Activist History Project.* Toronto, ON. Retrieved from https://aidsactivisthistory.files.wordpress.com/2016/06/aahp_-_julia_barnett.pdf

Berlant, L. (2006). "Cruel optimism." *differences*, 17(3), 20–36.

Brown, G. (2014). "Interview by Alexis Shotwell and Gary Kinsman." *AIDS Activist History Project.* Toronto, ON. Retrieved from https://aidsactivisthistory.files.wordpress.com/2016/06/aahp_-_glen_brown.pdf

Burke, K. (1984). *Permanence and change: An anatomy of purpose* (3rd ed.). Berkeley, CA: University of California Press.

Chambers, R. (2001). *Facing it: AIDS diaries and the death of the author.* Ann Arbor, MI: University of Michigan Press.

Code, L. (2006). *Ecological thinking: The politics of epistemic location.* Oxford/New York: Oxford University Press.

Conrad, R., & Shotwell, A. (2018). "'This is my body': Historical trauma, activist perfor-mance and embodied rage." *a/b: Auto/Biography Studies*, 33(2), 449–453.

de Montigny, G. (2017). "Ethnomethodological indifference: Just a passing phase?" *Human Studies*, 40(3): 331–364.

Dubriwny, T.N. (2012). *The vulnerable empowered woman: Feminism, postfeminism, and women's health.* New Brunswick, NJ: Rutgers University Press.

du Plessis, R. (2014). "Interview by Alexis Shotwell and Gary Kinsman." *AIDS Activist History Project.* Toronto, ON. Retrieved from https://aidsactivisthistory.files.wordpress.com/2016/06/aahp_-_renee_du_plessis.pdf

Ellingson, L. (2015). "Embodied practices in dialysis care: On (para)professional work." In B. Green and N. Hopwood (Eds.). *The body in professional practice* (pp. 73–189). Swit-zerland: Springer.

Emmons, K. (2009). *Black dogs and blue words: Depression and gender in the age of self-care.* New Brunswick, NJ: Rutgers University Press.

Garland-Thomson, R. (2007). "Shape structures story: Fresh and feisty stories about dis-ability." *Narrative*, 15(1), 113–123.

Garland-Thomson, R. (2015). "A habitable world: Harriet McBryde Johnson's 'case for my life'." *Hypatia*, 30(1), 300–306.

George, A., & Selzer, J. (2007). *Kenneth Burke in the 1930s*. Columbia, SC: University of South Carolina Press.

Hensley Owens, K. (2015). *Writing childbirth: Women's rhetorical agency in labor and online*. Carbondale, IL: Southern Illinois University Press.

Kinsman, G. (2014). "Interview by Alexis Shotwell." *AIDS Activist History Project*. Toronto, ON. Retrieved from https://aidsactivisthistory.files.wordpress.com/2016/06/aahp_-_gary_kinsman.pdf

Kinsman, G. (2018). "AIDS Activism: Remembering resistance versus socially organized forgetting." In S. Hindmarch, M. Orsini, & M. Gagnon (Eds.). *Seeing red: HIV/AIDS and public policy in Canada* (pp. 311–333). Toronto, ON: University of Toronto Press.

Klostermann, J. (2018). "Art, ordinary work and conceptuality: Sculpting the social relations of the art world." *Ethnography and Education*. Retrieved from www.tandfonline.com/toc/reae20/current

Loyd, J.M. (2014). *Health rights are civil rights: Peace and justice activism in Los Angeles, 1963–1978*. Minneapolis, MN: University of Minnesota Press.

McCaskell, T. (2014). "Interview by Alexis Shotwell and Gary Kinsman." *AIDS Activist History Project*. Toronto, ON. Retrieved from https://aidsactivisthistory.files.wordpress.com/2016/06/aahp_-_timmccaskell.pdf

Miller, C.R., & Shepherd, D. (2004). "Blogging as social action: A genre analysis of the weblog." In L. Gurak, S. Antonijevic, L. Johnson, C. Ratliff, & J. Reyman (Eds.). *Into the blogosphere: Rhetoric, community, and culture of weblogs*. Minnesota, MN: University of Minnesota. Retrieved from http://hdl.handle.net/11299/172818

Mykhalovskiy, E. (2014). "Interview by Alexis Shotwell and Gary Kinsman." *AIDS Activist History Project*. Toronto, ON. Retrieved from https://aidsactivisthistory.files.wordpress.com/2016/06/aahp_-_eric_mykhalovskiy.pdf

Restaino, J. (2015). "Surrender as method: Research, writing, rhetoric, love." *Peitho Journal*, 18(1): 72–95.

Rice, C., & Mündell, I. (2018). "Story-making as methodology: Disrupting dominant stories through multimedia storytelling." *CRS/RCS*, 55(2): 211–231.

Rich, A. (1972). "When we dead awaken: Writing as re-vision." *College English*, 34(1):18–30.

Scott, J.B. (2003). *Risky rhetoric: AIDS and the cultural practices of HIV testing*. Urbana, IL: Southern Illinois University Press.

Sedgwick, E.K. (2006). *Tendencies*. Durham, NC: Duke University Press.

Segal, J.Z. (2012). "Cancer experience and its narration: An accidental study." *Literature and Medicine*, 30(2): 292–318.

Segal, J.Z. (2015). "The rhetoric of female sexual dysfunction: Faux feminism and the FDA." *CMAJ Humanities*, 187(12): 915–916.

Selzer, J. (1999). "Habeas corpus: An introduction." In J. Selzer & S. Crowley (Eds.). *Rhetorical bodies* (pp. 3–15). Madison, WI: University of Wisconsin Press.

Shotwell, A. (2013). "Aspirational solidarity as bioethical norm: The case of reproductive justice." *IJFAB: International Journal of Feminist Approaches to Bioethics*, 6(1): 103–120.

Shotwell, A. (2016a). *Against purity: Living ethically in compromised times*. Minneapolis, MN: University of Minnesota Press.

Shotwell, A. (2016b). "Fierce love: What we can learn about epistemic responsibility from histories of AIDS advocacy." *Feminist Philosophy Quarterly*, 2(2): 1–16.

Siegel Finer, B. (2016). "The rhetoric of previving: Blogging the breast cancer gene." *Rhetoric Review*, 35(2): 176–188.

Smith, D.E. (2005). *Institutional ethnography: A sociology for people*. London: Rowman Altamira.

Smith, G.W. (n.d.). "Rites: Talking politics by George Smith: Police shape politics of AIDS." *AIDS Activist History Project.* Toronto, ON. Retrieved from https://aidsacti visthistory.omeka.net/items/show/627

Southin, B. (2014). "Interview by Alexis Shotwell and Gary Kinsman." *AIDS Activist History Project.* Toronto, ON. Retrieved from https://aidsactivisthistory.files.wordpress. com/2016/06/aahp_-_brent_southin.pdf

Sri. (2014). "Interview with Robin Turney by Alexis Shotwell and Gary Kinsman." *AIDS Activist History Project.* Toronto, ON. Retrieved from https://aidsactivisthistory.files. wordpress.com/2016/06/aahp-robin-turney-sri.pdf

Stenberg, S. (2006). "Making room for new subjects: Feminist interruptions of critical pedagogy rhetorics." In K. Ronald & J.S. Ritchie (Eds.). *Teaching rhetorica: Theory, pedagogy, practice* (pp. 131–146). Portsmouth, NH: Boynton/Cook.

Stenberg, S. (2018). "Tweet me your first assaults: Writing shame and the rhetorical work of #NotOkay." *Rhetoric Society Quarterly,* 48(2): 119–138.

Taylor, D. (2014). "Interview by Alexis Shotwell and Gary Kinsman." *AIDS Activist History Project.* Toronto, ON. Retrieved from https://aidsactivisthistory.files.wordpress. com/2016/06/aahp_-_darien_taylor.pdf

Waite, S. (2015). "Cultivating the scavenger: A queerer feminist future for composition and rhetoric." *Peitho,* 18(1): 51–71.

"Women get AIDS" (n.d.) Pamphlet. *AIDS Activist History Project Archives.* Retrieved from: https://aidsactivisthistory.omeka.net/items/show/22

15

COSTLY EXPEDIENCE

Reproductive Rights and Responses to Slut Shaming

Laurie McMillan

At the end of February 2012, Georgetown law student Sandra Fluke testified before Congress on behalf of women's right to free contraceptives under the ACA. Over the course of a few days, radio talk show host Rush Limbaugh responded on his show by labeling Fluke a "slut" who wanted taxpayers to pay for her to engage in unlimited sex (Wemple, 2012). Negative publicity ensued in reaction to Limbaugh, and approximately 40 of his sponsors withdrew their support. Although his network reiterated its support of him, Limbaugh chose to issue an apology.

This series of exchanges provides a lens into the ways rhetorics of slut-shaming and reproductive rights often intersect. "Slut-shaming" refers to the use of the label "slut" to marginalize a girl or woman by damaging her reputation with implications of overly sexual behavior (Bazelon, 2014, p. 95); such name-calling may be leveraged against women who have expressed sexual desire or against women who have not been sexually active but rather have challenged prescribed feminine norms (Duncan, 1999, p. 14). While Fluke's testimony largely sidesteps arguments about women's sexual behavior, Limbaugh draws on traditions of using slut-shaming to discredit women (in this case, Sandra Fluke) and to argue against reproductive rights (in this case, access to contraception). However, because his diatribe is leveled against a white law student at Georgetown University who does not fit typical stereotypes associated with the word "slut," Limbaugh faced extensive backlash.

I consider three public challenges to Limbaugh's comments to show why and how his narrative was ultimately rejected; after all, slut-shaming narratives are *not* often widely rejected. The responses to Limbaugh include a public statement from former Limbaugh sponsor David Friend, CEO of Carbonite; a satirical flowchart titled "Are You a Slut?" from the Mother Jones website (Murphy, &

Breedlove, 2012); and a YouTube video of the song "I'm a Slut" from the comedy duo the Reformed Whores. The responses argue that access to contraceptives affects so many women for such a variety of reasons that the word "slut" is inappropriate and unfair. However, because these responses reflect Fluke's social status and her minimal attention to women's sexual activity in her testimony, they may be limited in their ability to change long-term views about reproductive rights and women's sexuality. Looking closely at the rhetorics of the Fluke–Limbaugh controversy thus shows how short-term advocacy for reproductive rights may unintentionally compromise long-term progressive goals.

Slut-Shaming Narratives and Reproductive Rights

The Fluke–Limbaugh exchange and the ensuing backlash against Limbaugh are best understood in light of arguments against reproductive rights that center on women's sexuality. The most common anti-abortion arguments are framed as "pro-life"—as ethical obligations to protect unborn babies from murder (Lake, 1986, p. 482). However, as Lake (1984) explains, "anti-abortion rhetoric is not solely an attack on those who would violate [...] the moral proscription against killing, but also on those who would threaten Order in general via the sexual" (p. 433). In this framework, sexual desire is associated with immorality, and pregnancy is the price women are required to pay when they are promiscuous; the threat of this "punishment" (pregnancy) is meant to discourage excessive sexual activity (Lake, 1984, pp. 433–434). Others within the pro-life movement avoid the rhetoric of punishment by positioning themselves as pro-women. They focus on the emotional toll of abortions and suggest that women are often coerced into having abortions by unsupportive male partners (Moczulski, 2014, pp. 29–30). However, even when anti-abortion advocates claim they are speaking for the vulnerable and are not speaking "*against* women," proposed policies are often "straightforwardly punitive, imposing external authority and obligations upon women in an effort to control their irresponsible, immoral behavior and its consequences" (Lake, 1984, p. 434).

Lake's contentions that anti-abortion rhetoric is infused with concerns about promiscuity and sexual immorality are borne out in proposed government policies, politicians' public remarks, and anti-abortion literature. For example, Arduser and Koerber (2014) discuss politician Rick Santorum's position that sex should take place within marriage; therefore, contraception is dangerous and "*not* okay, because it's a license to do things in the sexual realm that is counter to how things are supposed to be" (p. 127). Similarly, the Concerned Women for America Legislative Action Committee published a "Pro-Life Action Guide" (2013) that shared stories of irresponsible women and overall social demise (2013, pp. 11–12). The guide described a woman who had nine abortions as if she is typical, and it argues that:

[Abortion] has corrupted romance and sexuality. In the ancient times before Roe, the price of an unwanted pregnancy could be terrifyingly high. That gave unmarried women a powerful incentive to be careful—to reserve themselves for men whom they knew to be worthy

(p. 11)

Baklinski and Bourne (2015) reference Cardinal Sean O'Malley's implication of the reverse cause-effect relationship by arguing that abortions would be less likely if "the promiscuous behavior that is rampant in our culture" were discouraged (para. 2). These arguments against reproductive freedoms rely on a heteronormative narrative of monogamy as they demonize sexual expression outside the setting of marriage.

Prescriptive judgments regarding sex, marriage, morality, and social demise can be considered an implicit form of slut-shaming that casts some people as immoral actors. When cultural narratives present sexual activity as immoral, the less powerful members of the culture tend to be associated with—and blamed for—that immorality. Arduser and Koerber (2014) explain that "antiabortion and anticontraception discourses" grant some people "full citizenship" while others are viewed as "citizens in need of surveillance as a means to protect them, as well as to protect the best interests of society" (p. 118). Explicit or implicit slut-shaming helps justify such inequities by reinforcing beliefs that "women's bodies and sexuality" are "dangerous, excessive, and difficult to control" (pp. 132–133). Longstanding double standards position sexually active or polyamorous women as dirty or immoral "sluts," while sexually active or polyamorous men are "studs." This double standard is reflected in ongoing attempts to police and legislate women's sexual behavior and reproductive choices.

As this double standard is challenged, some women tend to benefit more quickly than others. White, affluent, heterosexual women tend to be associated with sexual innocence (Egan, 2013, p. 136) and thus have some freedom to explore sexual options and challenge restrictive cultural narratives (Armstrong et al., 2014, p. 104). It is riskier for women of color, poor women, and others with less social capital to disrupt norms. Stereotypes depicting marginalized groups as unclean, tainted, immoral, and sexually promiscuous make it especially difficult for women of color and working-class women to challenge problematic ideas about sexual behavior (Egan, 2013, p. 17). Arguments about reproductive rights are further vexed for women of color because contraceptives and abortion have both been associated with eugenics and social resistance to miscegenation (Lombardo, 1996, pp. 23–25). While white women have long fought for the right to prevent or end pregnancy, women of color and poor women have fought for the right to bear children, and they continue to seek access to reproductive healthcare in the midst of a history of coerced sterilization and inadequate medical attention (Rutherford, 1992; see also Whitney, this collection).

Debates about reproductive freedoms are thus connected to issues of gender, race, class, and sex, even when advocates on either side try to reframe the issues and avoid discussing sex and morality. My contention is that long-term progressive change involves recognizing and challenging these underlying narratives. To the degree that arguments are reframed to become more widely accepted, some (white, heterosexual, affluent) women gain rights and freedoms while members of more vulnerable populations continue to struggle. At the same time, I recognize that leveraging less controversial arguments and advocating for gradual change can help cultural beliefs and practices evolve over time. The Fluke–Limbaugh controversy is a prime example of this tension. I first examine the rhetorics associated with Fluke's testimony and Limbaugh's response, then turn to three critiques of Limbaugh to evaluate their short-term and long-term advocacy potential around reproductive freedom.

Fluke, Limbaugh, and Women's Sexuality

In 2012, the Fluke–Limbaugh controversy at first seemed divorced from any discussion of women's sexual behavior. Democrats requested that Fluke speak to the House Oversight and Government Reform Committee during a discussion of the ACA. While the ACA allowed churches to refuse contraceptive coverage, religiously affiliated organizations (such as hospitals or schools) that employed people of various faith backgrounds were obligated to provide access to contraception. Conservatives proposed the Blunt Amendment, a "Conscience Clause" to exempt employers from this obligation, and Fluke objected.

The panel that actually assembled before the Oversight Committee did not include Fluke. Indeed, only men were included in the meeting, with the defense that the issue of access to contraceptives was one of religious freedom, an area in which Fluke lacked expertise (Legge et al., 2012, p. 175). Framing the debate as a question of religious freedom deferred attention to women's sexuality, even though the phrase "morally objectionable" implies that women's sexual and reproductive choices are the crux of the matter. Rather than forefront a debate about women's sexual activity in a culture where contraceptive use is widely accepted, both politicians and religious leaders emphasized religious rights and avoided discussion of contraceptives, sex, and morality. In other words, this argument could not proceed by emphasizing a "pro-life" moral imperative, so legislators crafted a narrative of vulnerable religious organizations—or even corporations with religious affiliations—being attacked and bullied by an intrusive and unethical government.

When Fluke was excluded from the Oversight Committee, she was invited to speak to the House Democratic Steering and Policy Committee. One might expect that Fluke would reveal and challenge the narrative framing of religious freedom by emphasizing the problem of judging and punishing women for having sex. Instead, she pointed out that religious freedoms were not being infringed upon with awareness that women are easily demonized for sexual activity. She played the same game as her opponents but from a different angle: She presented herself as a hardworking and humble student with very little power, and she told stories of responsible women who were unfairly denied access to contraceptives.

From the start, Fluke minimized her own voice in order to share the stories of others' suffering: "I want to thank you for allowing them—them, not me—to be heard" (Moorhead, 2012, para. 4). Fluke avoided being perceived as attention seeking, loud, pushy, or otherwise powerful. In the course of her testimony, she positioned women as "powerless" victims who are "suffering," carrying "burdens," and "struggling" in ways that their male counterparts are not (Moorhead, 2012, paras. 3–6). Fluke created a sense that the suffering is widespread by using statistics and offering logical reasons why contraception should be covered under the ACA. To a great degree, however, she relied on seven individual stories to showcase women's medical, financial, and emotional burdens. Most of the stories offered glimpses of women who face financial hardship, find themselves with impossible choices, are trying to be responsible and take care of their health, but face one barrier after another. Most of these women are married, with Fluke likely trying "to stave off criticisms that women just want to sleep around" (Moczulski, 2014, p. 37). The most extensive story told was of a woman with PCOS who faced intense medical problems (including the threat of infertility) when she couldn't afford the birth control she needed to treat her condition. These stories emphasized women who are victims of a sexist health system.

Although in his later apology, Limbaugh complained that "it is absolutely absurd that during these very serious political times, we are discussing personal sexual recreational activities before members of Congress" (Limbaugh, 2012b), Fluke's testimony did not discuss "personal sexual recreational activities" in any way. In fact, "sex" was not mentioned at all in Fluke's testimony, though "sexual" was used as a modifier when she told a story of a friend who was raped. Fluke never addressed Conservative concerns about sexual morality but instead worked to "lessen the audience's association of the Conscience Clause with sexual desire" (Moczulski, 2014, p. 37). Religious or moral exceptions to contraception are illogical in this framing. Focusing on married women and on the role of contraceptives for a variety of medical conditions allowed Fluke to appeal to listeners who may be predisposed to dismiss arguments supporting diverse sexual practices and the importance of contraception.

Because Fluke never discussed her own sex life or anyone else's sexual habits, Limbaugh's remarks misrepresent her testimony:

> Sandra Fluke, whatever her name is—the Georgetown student who went before a congressional committee and said she's having so much sex, she's going broke buying contraceptives and wants us to buy them. I said, "Well, what would you call someone who wants us to pay for her to have sex? What would you call that woman? You'd call 'em a slut, a prostitute or whatever."
>
> *(Limbaugh, 2012c)*

In the course of the above excerpted transcript, Limbaugh used the word "sex" 55 times in his denigration of Fluke and her support of contraception, with ten of those instances being phrased as "so much sex." Limbaugh used the term "slut" and the repeated mischaracterization of Fluke's testimony to recast an argument about women's equal access to healthcare into a narrative of immoral and irresponsible women taking advantage of hardworking taxpayers. Limbaugh's "extreme use of demeaning language" painted Fluke as someone with "loose morals" in "an attempt to demean any credibility that Fluke's testimony may have" (Moczulski, 2014, p. 49). Here, the person fighting for rights (that is, Fluke) is represented as the "bad guy" who is actually trying to disadvantage others. That is exactly the way the word "slut" often operates: it recasts people being treated unfairly (through name-calling and the repercussions of such negative labeling) as people who are unworthy and who are themselves engaged in bad and hurtful behavior (Walter-Bailey, & Goodman, 2005). Often, then, the "slut" label makes victims look like aggressors.

Limbaugh's response to Fluke exposed a narrative of sex and reproductive rights that already existed but had remained an unspoken undercurrent, whether in claims that access to contraception is solely a matter of religious freedom or in Fluke's focus on married women and medical conditions. Limbaugh thus simultaneously ignored actual testimony from Congress and exposed the elephant in the room: single women have sex, and some people are not okay with that. In fact, some people are so disturbed by the idea of single women having sex that Fluke does not even mention it. In the course of slut-shaming Fluke, Limbaugh also reiterates the idea that women who have sex ought to face "consequences": "We're told that people […] want to have sex without consequence, sex with no responsibility, and we have [to] pay for it!" (Limbaugh, 2012a). Limbaugh's remarks also show how the poor are more vulnerable to negative judgment when sex is believed to exert a cost on participants: "Well, have you ever thought maybe you shouldn't? If you can't afford it, you can't do it" (Limbaugh, 2012a). Such remarks are ignorant of the sexual nature of human beings as they view sex as a costly option to be enjoyed by men (who don't get pregnant) and the wealthy (who can afford birth control).

Slut-shaming is often an effective way of ostracizing and silencing a woman. In this situation, it had the opposite effect. Limbaugh's remarks were condemned, and Fluke received more attention, allowing her to continue advocating for access to contraception. To better understand why Limbaugh's attempt to slut shame Fluke failed and the larger implications of this debate, I consider the impact of the rhetorical choices in three responses to his remarks.

Costly Expedience: Three Sample Responses

Considering a range of responses to the controversy Limbaugh created for himself suggests that one of his key mistakes was slut-shaming the wrong person. Fluke's social status and her focus on medical rather than sexual themes made it easy for the wider public to take her side in the debate. Because sponsors withdrew from Limbaugh's radio show and because Limbaugh was eventually compelled to apologize to Fluke, the responses to his slut-shaming seem successful. However, the short-term success may be due to continued avoidance of difficult questions about sex, morality, and exactly who in our culture is considered worthy of support. To explore the tension between short-term expedient advocacy and long-term progressive goals, I consider three increasingly progressive responses to Limbaugh.

The first and least progressive of these is a public statement issued by David Friend, CEO of Carbonite, a company that had advertised during Limbaugh's show. Friend wrote:

> No one with daughters the age of Sandra Fluke, and I have two, could possibly abide the insult and abuse heaped upon this courageous and well-intentioned young lady. Mr. Limbaugh, with his highly personal attacks on Miss Fluke, overstepped any reasonable bounds of decency. Even though Mr. Limbaugh has now issued an apology, we have nonetheless decided to withdraw our advertising from his show. We hope that our action, along with the other advertisers who have already withdrawn their ads, will ultimately contribute to a more civilized public discourse.
>
> *(Friend, 2012, para. 1)*

This response presents Fluke as a person who deserves chivalry. She is "Miss Fluke," a "courageous and well-intentioned" "young lady," and the speaker calls for "decency" and "civilized public discourse." Friend shows a gentlemanly respect for Sandra Fluke that condemns Limbaugh's approach as much by contrast as by criticism. This response is aligned with findings that people are more likely to oppose an action if the victim of the offense—in this case, Sandra Fluke—seems to be "dignified, honorable, or noble"—attributes that render the offense less justifiable (Legge et al., 2012, pp. 180–181).

Fluke's "honorable" status is further exemplified by the paternalism of Friend's explanation. Because Fluke is similar to his daughters, he responds like a father who should protect her from Limbaugh's inappropriate commentary. Friend's ability to relate to Fluke is helpful in one sense: if we can imagine people who are being hurt as similar to people we care about, we are more likely to take action on their behalf. On the other hand, this approach may ultimately be problematic. If Sandra Fluke were very different from David Friend's daughters, would he still respond to her sympathetically? What if she were older, of a different ethnicity or race, less educated, poor, or male? In short, it seems like a fine idea to respond to an incident ethically by finding ways to care about the actors involved, but it seems short-sighted to have such caring rely on the similarity to one's own family or immediate community.

The other two sample responses use satire to challenge Limbaugh's slut-shaming and thus operate differently from Friend's statement. A flowchart by Tim Murphy and Ben Breedlove (2012) titled "Are You a Slut?" (see Figure 15.1) exposes the double standards used by Limbaugh and his supporters. The flowchart starts with a red box asking, "Do you ever have sex for, like, non-procreative reasons?" with the informal language signaling the playful and ironic tone. There are three possible outcomes for the flowchart (each in white). The only way a woman can avoid being a slut is by having sex only for procreation, not using birth control (even for medical reasons) and believing that women who use birth control are sluts. Any other choices lead a woman to be a slut. Men, on the other hand, are never sluts. No matter how a man answers the questions, the flowchart ends with "Of course you're not a slut; you're a dude! Rock on, bro!" One of the questions sarcastically alludes to Limbaugh's criminal charge of carrying Viagra prescribed to someone else *en route* to a bachelor party.

The flowchart clearly and humorously depicts a double standard that casts women as "sluts" on a regular basis while male sexuality is affirmed. It highlights illogical and inconsistent judgments—both the irony of Limbaugh criticizing Fluke *and* the more general problem when women are considered sluts simply because they're women who think it is appropriate for other women to use contraceptives or do so themselves. The flowchart is contextualized with an introduction that briefly summarizes the way Fluke was inappropriately "maligned for oversharing about her sex life, which she didn't even discuss on the Hill" (Murphy, & Breedlove, 2012). The flowchart thus goes much further in exposing the way the word "slut" operates on an unjust gendered basis than David Friend's remarks do.

The flowchart works because most people would find it ridiculous to call a woman a slut because she uses contraception. The chart would likely be less effective if it addressed other behaviors associated with slut-shaming, such as women having multiple partners, openly expressing sexual desire, or calling attention to themselves. These kinds of extended arguments against slut-shaming are important for disrupting Rush Limbaugh's extremism, blatantly sexist cultural narratives, and religious traditions that negatively affect many women, especially poor women and women of color (Guttmacher Institute, 2016; Howell, & Starrs, 2017). While the flowchart is more effective than David Friend's public statement in its challenge to Limbaugh's sexist double standard, its argument relies on adherence to widely accepted beliefs that may not be helpful in advocating for reproductive freedoms beyond this particular question of access to contraceptives.

Another satirical response to Limbaugh's vitriol, the Reformed Whores (2012) song "I'm a Slut," combines specifics from the political moment with additional critiques of misogynist social attitudes. The song was recorded as a YouTube video and was widely shared during the Limbaugh–Fluke controversy. It now has over 500,000 views. The video juxtaposes traditional elements of non-threatening femininity with progressive views of women and sexuality, to some degree paralleling

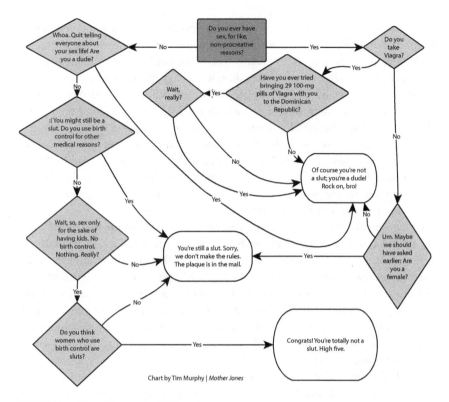

FIGURE 15.1 "Are You a Slut?" flowchart

Sandra Fluke's presentation as a self-effacing and noble advocate for responsible women facing financial hardships in their quests for adequate medical care.

In the video, the comedic duo the Reformed Whores, Katy Frame and Marie Cecile Anderson, appear neatly groomed in old-fashioned pastel-colored dresses with ruffles and thus seem aligned with conservative ideals of femininity. The women play an accordion and ukulele to provide country and western style music, a genre associated with traditional conservative values. The women dance in goofy ways during the video, adding to the implicit message that these women are not sexual, attention-seeking, or otherwise associated with slut stereotypes.

The song begins by describing teens who call their promiscuous peers "sluts." The chorus then argues that Limbaugh has "redefined" the term, so it can now be used for a person who is educated, responsible, and who speaks up. This general description clearly refers to Fluke and other women like her. The next two verses identify even more women who would be considered sluts according to Limbaugh's use of the word, including a married woman who has only had sex with her husband and uses birth control for family planning, as well as a teen who was prescribed birth control because of menstrual discomfort. These examples highlight how ludicrous Limbaugh's response to Fluke is, especially because in her testimony, she specifically referenced the importance of contraceptives for these purposes.

These parts of the song are similar to the flowchart because in their focus on challenging Limbaugh's remarks, they do not really challenge the practice of slut-shaming more generally. However, the Reformed Whores extend the claim by saying if a teen girl wants to have sex, it's no one's business outside of the private relationship. Here, the initial definition of a slut as a teenager who has had sex with more than one partner is slightly dismantled. The Reformed Whores thus *do* attempt to show how the term "slut" has been applied widely by Limbaugh and how even the more typical use of the term is inappropriate. They also deconstruct resistance to educated women by calling themselves snobs and elitists, again using satire to point out the absurdity of such accusations.

To sum up, David Friend's response suggests that no woman can be labeled a slut who is similar to his daughters. Although it is certainly unintentional, such conflation suggests that it is unacceptable for only white, affluent, well-educated, well-groomed, professional women to be labeled sluts. Murphy's flowchart goes further in implying that having sex and using birth control should not be condemned. By responding specifically to the Fluke–Limbaugh controversy, however, the flowchart leaves the most typical uses of the "slut" label—and its implications for reproductive rights—unacknowledged and unaddressed. Finally, the Reformed Whores video uses the Limbaugh controversy to both comment on his inappropriate comments toward Fluke and address the policing of the sexual behavior of teen girls and resentment of well-educated women. They present women as complex and resist labels by combining a conservative style with progressive and slightly racy lyrics. They move in the direction of challenging the connections between sexual behavior, morality, and reproductive rights.

After Effects

When people rejected Limbaugh's attempts to slut shame Fluke, the short-term effect was that Limbaugh apologized and walked back his remarks. The ACA kept a provision that women could access free birth control via insurers if employers held moral objections to contraception, with the likelihood that Limbaugh's remarks contributed to the failure of arguments that framed the debate as a question of religious freedom (Legge et al., 2012, p. 199). The negative response to Limbaugh might have helped raise awareness that slut-shaming is inappropriate (p. 197), though there's a risk that the actual lesson learned was that slut-shaming (white, educated) women (who possess a lot of social capital) is inappropriate. Additionally, the backlash against Limbaugh may have contributed to Romney's loss in the 2012 presidential election due to its association with a "Republican War on Women" (Legge et al., 2012, p. 194).

However, at the state level, reproductive freedoms have continued to be challenged with legislative restrictions (Arduser and Koerber, 2014, p. 133). For example, a Guttmacher Institute report on state policies in the first quarter of 2018 included information about eight states expanding access to reproductive health services while five states "adopted 10 new abortion restrictions" and 37 states "[introduced] 347 measures to restrict access to either abortion or contraception" (Nash et al., 2018, para. 2). Some of the restrictions "ban abortion under certain circumstances" such as a "specified point in pregnancy"; some require abortion clinics to provide extensive reports of any complications that arise, and some legislate specific counseling that women are required to receive before and after abortion procedures (Nash et al., 2018). This is just a small sampling of state policies enacted in just three months.

Although continued attacks on reproductive freedoms cannot be blamed on the Fluke–Limbaugh controversy, I do think there was a missed opportunity to directly refute the belief that women's sexual behaviors and desires are immoral. Republicans and religious leaders tried to sidestep that conversation and Fluke joined them. When Limbaugh gave voice to the slut-shaming narratives that underlie opposition to reproductive rights, he exposed the offensiveness and misogyny that are often clothed in rhetorics of concern about women, social demise, or a loss of family values.

Imagine if David Friend had amended his remarks to say that even women who do not resemble his daughters should not be called sluts. Imagine if his daughters spoke up, noting that many women who are more vulnerable than they are deserve respect and should have control of their healthcare choices. Imagine if the flowchart challenged Limbaugh's hypocrisy and the phrase "Conscience Clause" by suggesting that punishing women for having sex is not a sign of morality but is rather a sign of twisted repression. The Reformed Whores make the boldest move to address problematic assumptions about sexual behavior that guides thinking about reproductive health. To be clear, all three responses deserve credit for taking increasingly risky positions as they addressed the controversy. Yet, I believe the short-term goals of defending Fluke and her argument for access to contraception could have been accomplished while *also* fully challenging broader slut-shaming narratives that are still used to justify control of women's bodies and restrictive reproductive policies.

References

Arduser, L., & Koerber, A. (2014). "Splitting women, producing biocitizens, and vilifying Obamacare in the 2012 presidential campaign." *Women's Studies in Communication*, 37(2), 117–137.

Armstrong, E.A., Hamilton, L.T., Armstrong, E.M., & Seeley, J.L. (2014). "'Good Girls' gender, social class, and slut discourse on campus." *Social Psychology Quarterly*, 77(2), 100–122.

Baklinski, P., & Bourne, L. (2015). "'Glamorization of promiscuity' must end before abortion can, cardinal O'Malley tells 11,000 at March for Life Vigil." Retrieved from www.life sitenews.com/news/glamorization-of-promiscuity-must-end-before-abortion-can-cardina l-omalley

Bazelon, E. (2014). *Sticks and stones: Defeating the culture of bullying and rediscovering the power of character and empathy.* New York: Random House.

Concerned Women for America Legislative Action Committee. (2013). "Pro-life action guide: Upholding truth, protecting life." Retrieved from http://concernedwomen.org/wp-content/uploads/2013/11/pro-life.pdf

Duncan, N. (1999). *Sexual bullying: Gender conflict and pupil culture in secondary schools.* New York: Routledge.

Egan, R.D. (2013). *Becoming sexual: A critical appraisal of the sexualization of girls.* New York: John Wiley & Sons.

Friend, D. (2012). "A statement from David Friend, CEO of Carbonite." In Facebook [Carbonite Business Page]. Retrieved May 4, 2018 from www.facebook.com/Carboni teOnlineBackup/posts/a-statement-from-david-friend-ceo-of-carboniteno-one-with-da ughters-the-age-of-s/10150573840040976/

Guttmacher Institute (2016). "U.S. intended pregnancy rate falls to 30-year low; declines seen in almost all groups, but disparities remain." Retrieved from www.guttmacher.org/news-relea se/2016/us-unintended-pregnancy-rate-falls-30-year-low-declines-seen-almost-all-groups

Howell, M., & Starrs, A.M. (2017). "For women of color, access to vital health services is threatened." Retrieved from https://thehill.com/blogs/pundits-blog/healthcare/ 343996-for-women-of-color-access-to-vital-health-services-is

Lake, R.A. (1986). "The metaethical framework of anti-abortion rhetoric." *Signs: Journal of Women in Culture and Society,* 11(3), 478–499.

Lake, R.A. (1984). "Order and disorder in anti-abortion rhetoric: A logological view." *Quarterly Journal of Speech,* 70(4), 425–443.

Legge, N.J., DiSanza, J.R., Gribas, J., & Shiffler, A. (2012). "'He sounded like a vile, disgusting pervert …': An analysis of persuasive attacks on Rush Limbaugh during the Sandra Fluke controversy." *Journal of Radio & Audio Media,* 19(2), 173–205.

Limbaugh, R. (2012a). "A statement from Rush [Radio Series Episode]." In The Rush Limbaugh Show. Premier Radio Network. West Palm Beach, FL. Retrieved from www.rushlimbaugh.com/daily/2012/03/03/a_statement_from_rush/

Limbaugh, R. (2012b). "The Democrats are desperate: Obama calls Sandra Fluke, the 30-year-old victim [Radio Series Episode]." In The Rush Limbaugh Show. Premier Radio Network. West Palm Beach, FL. Retrieved from www.rushlimbaugh.com/daily/2012/ 03/02/the_democrats_are_desperate_obama_calls_sandra_fluke_the_30_year_old_victim/

Limbaugh, R. (2012c, March 1). "X – Left freaks out over my fluke remarks [Radio Series Episode]." In The Rush Limbaugh Show. Premier Radio Network. West Palm Beach, FL. Retrieved from www.rushlimbaugh.com/daily/2012/03/01/x_left_freaks_out_ over_my_fluke_remarks

Lombardo, P.A. (1996). "Medicine, eugenics, and the Supreme Court: From coercive sterilization to reproductive freedom." *Journal of Contemporary Health Law and Policy,* 13(1), 1–25.

Moczulski, L.A. (2014). "Exploring the polyvocal leadership problem in the pro-life movement: The case of Rush Limbaugh and Sandra Fluke." [Doctoral dissertation]. Retrieved from https://wakespace.lib.wfu.edu/bitstream/handle/10339/39288/Moc zulski_wfu_0248M_10572.pdf

Moorhead, M. (2012). "In context: Sandra Fluke on contraceptives and women's health." Retrieved from www.politifact.com/truth-o-meter/article/2012/mar/06/context-sa ndra-fluke-contraceptives-and-womens-hea/

Murphy, T., & Breedlove, B. (2012). "Flowchart: Are you a slut?" Retrieved from www. motherjones.com/politics/2012/03/flow-chart-are-you-slut/

Nash, E., Mohammed, L., Ansari-Thomas, Z., Capello, O., & Benson Gold, R. (2018). "Policy trends in the states: First quarter 2018." Retrieved from www.guttmacher.org/a rticle/2018/04/policy-trends-states-first-quarter-2018

Reformed Whores. (2012). "Rush Limbaugh calls Sandra Fluke a slut—Reformed Whores' response video." [YouTube] Retrieved from www.youtube.com/watch?v=fZK75pXLlbY

Rutherford, C. (1992). "Reproductive freedom and African American women." *Yale Journal of Law and Feminism*, 4(2), 255–290.

Walter-Bailey, W., & Goodman, J. (2005). "Exploring the culture of 'sluthood' among adolescents." In S. Steinberg, P. Parmar, & B. Richard (Eds.). *Contemporary youth culture: An international encyclopedia* (pp. 280–283). Santa Barbara, CA: Greenwood ABC-CLIO.

Wemple, E. (2012, March 5). "Rush Limbaugh's 'personal attack' on Sandra Fluke? More like 20 attacks." Retrieved from www.washingtonpost.com/blogs/erik-wemp le/post/rush-limbaughs-personal-attack-on-sandra-fluke-more-like-20-attacks/2012/ 03/04/gIQA1OkHtR_blog.html?utm_term=.9171feeb4aff

AFTERWORD

"The Rhetorician [of Health and Medicine] as Agent of Social Change": Activism for the Whole Woman's Body

Bryna Siegel Finer

In 1996, Parrot and Condit edited *Evaluating Women's Health Messages: A Resource Book*. Perhaps the most comprehensive collection on women's health discourse, the volume contains 28 chapters on reproductive health and what has been referred to as "bikini-medicine": "concentrating on the breasts and the reproductive organs, while essentially ignoring the rest of the woman" (Gulati, 2017). In their introduction, the editors acknowledge this gap in their book, a focus that "can perpetuate problems for women [because] it may perpetuate the tendency to treat women as distinctive and important only because of their reproductive capacities" (Parrot, & Condit, 1996, p. 3). The editors had two goals for their book: "(a) identify gaps in research about women's health; and (b) identify gaps in messages about women's health" (p. 2). While their collection most certainly accomplished these goals in terms of reproductive health, we have a ways to go in other areas of women's health, especially in terms of illnesses that most often lead to women's deaths: heart disease, lung cancer, diabetes, and Alzheimer's. With the exception of Arduser's (2017) *Living Chronic: Agency and Expertise in the Rhetoric of Diabetes*, there is practically no RHM work in these areas of women's health. Like Dubriwny (2013), we, the co-editors of this collection, wanted to "revitalize the role of a feminist perspective on women's health, as the perspective offered by the women's health movement has been lost of misconstrued by the public and by medical researchers" (p. 2). We envisioned our collection building on Parrot and Condit's, yet moving beyond bikini medicine.

In reading the present collection as a whole, I can't help but wonder if scholars and researchers in rhetoric, communication, and similar disciplines have used the past 20+ years to make great strides in analyses of women's health messages and to wonder what application has been done with those analyses to improve the state of women's health. This book has much to offer, but it seems as if perhaps we've made only modest gains. For instance, we (women) know that we (women) are treated differently—and by differently, I mean poorly—by healthcare providers. Read any chapter in this book, and you'll see this evidence bear out again and again. And, although our current collection includes chapters on lupus, AIDS, and women's running injuries, it is still primarily focused on bikini-medicine; that is, it is focused on "sex-specific conditions that [only] affect women: breast and ovarian cancers, pregnancy, and menstrual cycles" (Women's Brain Health Initiative, 2015).

So, what have we done in this volume other than collect more evidence of what we already know? This important question is addressed in the introduction to the collection, where White-Farnham and Molloy acknowledge that "this work only begins to skim the surface of deeply troubling issues that need much more attention" (p. 000, this collection); yet they note that the collection overall "demonstrates the resolve of women who create change for themselves and others" (p. 000, this collection). Still, other important questions remain: why does it matter that women are treated badly in the US healthcare system and beyond, and what can those of us in RHM do about it?

Why Does it Matter How Women are Treated by Healthcare Providers? or, Why the Conversation About Women's Health Must Move Beyond the Bikini

Most women in the US die from heart disease, lung cancer, and Alzheimer's disease. But, and I admit I am just guessing here, I bet if I asked a random person on the street what they think most women die from, they would say breast cancer. Why? Because the US has been "pinkwashed," a term coined by Breast Cancer Action to signify:

> the significant lack of accountability, the absence of transparency, and the widespread hypocrisy in the pink ribbon marketing culture [that] exploits a disease that devastates communities, misrepresents who is affected by breast cancer, and excludes and marginalizes women's diverse lived experiences of the disease.
>
> *(Breast Cancer Action, 2019)*

Pink is on car bumpers, it's on NFL apparel (National Football League, 2015), it's on drill bits for hydraulic fracturing (Sartor, 2015). Pink is pervasive, and because of pink, people are more aware of breast cancer than ever (Parthasarathy, 2014). On the other hand, seven times the number of women die annually from heart disease than from breast cancer, yet 76% of women do not know their own cholesterol, and approximately 45% of women have cholesterol high enough to lead to heart attack or stroke (Centers for Disease Control, 2017). Yes, over 40,000 women die from breast cancer each year (American Cancer Society,

2019a), and that is 40,000 women too many. None of this is to say that we should not care about breast cancer, nor the women who suffer from or die from it. The issue is that the pink ribbon has become so rhetorically powerful that every woman I know has been persuaded by it, feeling the fear of it to their core, willing to do anything it tells them to do. This is not to set up a competition of diseases—which disease is harder for the patient, which is worse to suffer through? This—the fact that women are enculturated into a discourse in which breast cancer is omnipresent—is a rhetorical and embodied problem that causes women to needlessly suffer.

I know this personally. Like Dean (in this collection), I am BRCA positive, which means I am at high-risk for breast and ovarian cancer. After a diagnosis of DCIS (Stage 0 breast cancer, or pre-cancer) at age 36, I underwent a bilateral mastectomy, hysterectomy, and oophorectomy. Removal of the ovaries can reduce risk of breast cancer by 50% or more in premenopausal women (American Cancer Society, 2019b). Yet, the younger a woman is when her ovaries are removed, the more at-risk she becomes for coronary heart disease, hypertension, and cardiac arrhythmias (North American Menopause Society, 2018). Because I was (and still am) so afraid of breast cancer, I willingly put myself at an even higher risk for heart disease than a woman in the general population, which is already 1 in 4 (Centers for Disease Control, 2017). I have high cholesterol man-aged with medication. I also take medication for migraines that could cause a heart episode. Yet, when the radiologist showed me the scans of my right breast, and a few days later when the oncologist told me I should have my breasts and ovaries removed because of my BRCA status, I couldn't schedule the surgeries fast enough; within six months, nearly every bit that made me a biologically sexed woman was removed from my body. Why am I more scared of breast cancer than heart disease? Or, how did breast cancer become, arguably, the most rhetorically powerful illness known to (wo)mankind when we are seemingly unaffected by that which is much more likely to actually kill us? That is a ques-tion that feminist rhetoricians in health and medicine could be investigating.

More disconcerting, what should scare any woman like me the most about our risk of heart disease has nothing to do with lack of ovaries or high cholesterol. If I experience symptoms of a heart attack, I am quite likely not to be diagnosed as such; a doctor is likely to suggest I am having a panic attack, that I have acid reflux, or that I have some other issue *only because I am a woman*. A recent study showed that more than 50% of the time, doctors misdiagnose women's heart attack symptoms (Lichtman et al., 2018). These were women who went to their doctors with symptoms such as palpitations and arm pain, were told by their doctors they were fine, and then ended up in hospital with what could have been a preventable heart episode. Multiple other studies spanning the last two decades have shown similar results (see, for example, Yong, 2018; Spatz et. al., 2015; Anand et. al., 2005). This sexism, like pinkwashing, is a material reality, yet it is also a rhetorical and discursive phenomenon; this discourse is being studied by medical researchers, but not as frequently by those in RHM. Surely, there is much we can add to this conversation in order to improve conditions. So why does it matter how women are treated by healthcare providers? Because too many doctors do not take women's health seriously, and too many public discourses suggest that women's health does get plenty of attention, but that attention is disproportionately on bikini medicine. And then women die.

What Do We Do About the Way Women Are Treated by Healthcare Providers?

This afterword takes its title from the influential article, "Rhetorician as Agent of Social Change," in which Cushman (1996) describes, among other things, writing documents such as, "resumes, job applications, college applications, and dialogic journals ... recommendations to landlords, courts, potential employers, admissions counselors, and DSS representatives" (p. 13) with/for a community local to her university as part of and as reciprocation for their participation in her dissertation study. Cushman (1996) reminds rhetoricians that "in doing our scholarly work, we should take social responsibility for the people from whom we come to understand a topic" (p. 12). While compiling the chapters in this book, my co-editors and I had many discussions about the people herein and their material realities, especially the patients and study participants. What is our social responsibility to them? And are we fulfilling it in this scholarly work? Is developing this book—a book that offers yet more evidence of the tacit and overt forms of sexism in women's healthcare, even along with the strategies feminist activists use to contend with these challenging and often life-threatening realities—really enough? Where do we take this work, and how do we apply it to improve women's healthcare situations?

Readers of the present collection can learn a lot about how women are enacting vernacular health activism, often in the contexts of extremely daunting circumstances. However, there are also takeaways for rhetoricians of health and medicine for moving forward as we think about the literacy practices and rhetorical strategies described within by (and often about) some of these patients and patient-advocates. Here, I'd like to consider how these practices and strategies not only serve as examples of "scholarly activism, which facilitates the literate activities that already take place in the community" (Cushman, 1996, p. 13) as applied specifically to communities of female patients who have, historically, been treated with malfeasance, but also demonstrate ways that RHM "recognizes rhetoric as constitutive action" (Scott & Melonçon, 2018, p. 5).

As women are told repeatedly, and as this book evidences, if we want to be treated well in healthcare settings, we must be good self-advocates (see especially Dean, Laux, and Tadros in this collection); however, self-advocacy, when it comes to healthcare, is more than having an empowered voice. When it comes to healthcare, self-advocacy requires an empowered voice *backed by* literate practices and rhetorical strategies. In other words, reading and writing are necessary for literal survival.

My own healthcare experiences have taught me this important lesson in effective women's health advocacy. Although my mastectomy and other surgeries were six years ago, there have been residual effects. One of these has been chronic, excruciating back pain, which I've experienced for almost two years—most likely due to abdominal muscle weakness from reconstruction after the mastectomy. I've visited my primary care physician, my rheumatologist, two pain specialists, a back surgeon, an orthopedist, and three different physical therapists for a total of over 100 medical appointments; received two steroid injections between L4 and L5 in my spine, one in my sacroiliac joint, one in the trochanteric bursa of my hip, one in my ischial tuberosity, and one directly into my S1 nerve root; had two MRIs of my back, one of my pelvis, and one of my hip; and spent over $5,000 dollars in co-pays and deductibles, plus almost $2,000 on physical therapy not covered by insurance. After all this, an alternative medicine practitioner suggested I try an anti-inflammatory, but he would not prescribe it. My rheumatologist, however, did. I took the pill each night, and it allowed me to sleep well and wake up pain-free, but the pain returned midmorning; I counted the minutes until I could take my nightly dose. So, I went online. I read about the prescription on the pharmaceutical company website. I read about it on WebMD and asked some questions in a forum for patients with my condition. I went into my university library's PubMed database and read some journal articles about the efficacy and side-effects of the medication in various clinical trials. I used all of that information to make a decision: I began to take the pill twice a day, and I felt transformed—nearly pain-free around the clock. After a few days, I emailed my doctor and explained the results of my experiment; I asked for a new prescription for double the dosage. He responded later that day to tell me he had sent the new prescription to the pharmacy, and he had scheduled me for blood work later in the month to check my kidney and liver function.

When I think about this situation, almost two years of it, and especially down to this last moment, I am highly aware of the literacy strategies and rhetorical knowledge I have at my disposal. I know how to find resources in a variety of places, including university library databases and medical research journals. I know how to evaluate sources for credibility and critique the agendas of sources like pharmaceutical companies, naturopathic doctors, and patients in forums who have had a variety of both positive and negative experiences. I can write to inform and persuade my audience (my doctor) by considering his level of knowledge of my case (he has seen me every 4–6 months for almost seven years), the amount of time he has to read my email, and his positionality (he is the head of rheumatology at a large university hospital, not a first-year resident). Importantly, in this situation, I was successful in acquiring what I needed for my health not only because of self-advocacy, but because that self-advocacy was backed by literate practices and rhetorical strategies.

I recognize, however, that my position as a woman who's benefited from advanced training in writing and rhetoric is relatively uncommon. While many other women, of course, are highly educated and/or simply have had life experiences that have led them to deep knowledge of the roles language and persuasion play in healthcare situations, having a background in RHM might make me especially capable of self-advocacy in healthcare. As we close this project, I find myself reflecting on what that means in terms of my responsibility to other women who do not have my training. Cushman (1996) pushes rhetoricians to consider empowerment as more than just knowing: "To empower, as I use it, means: a) to enable someone to achieve a goal by providing resources for them; b) to facilitate actions—particularly those associated with language and literacy; c) to lend our power or status to forward people's achievement" (p. 14). As feminist scholars in RHM, we have a responsibility to do the "scholarly activism" Cushman refers to by empowering other women in hard health situations. Many of the women in this book write about their participants' empowerment or their own feelings of empowerment, almost always after learning a piece of information vital to their health situation. But how is that empowerment, then, used to facilitate action?

For instance, after years of helping patients fight against discrimination before the Genetic Information Nondiscrimination Act (2008), FORCE staff developed a full smorgasbord of written templates that BRCA positive people can download to use when fighting with insurance claims for coverage of testing and procedures. Their website explains, "To assist our community with insurance denial appeals, FORCE has created sample insurance appeal letters on […] screening and preventive services indicated for the hereditary cancer community" (FORCE, 2019). Even further, FORCE is in the process of developing a program where peers who feel comfortably insurance-literate will assist members of the community with using these templates. As a rhetorician in health and medicine, knowing that rhetorical strategies and literate practices are my strong suit, and having worked with previvors as a group of study participants, this is one way I could use "scholarly activism" to give back to my community and to further advocate on behalf of its cause. In some ways, this is similar to the work Cushman did for her community of study participants. In this collection, McKinley mentions that, as part of her IRB process, she has offered to give her data to the facilitators of the patient discussion board she studied, thus providing them with knowledge that they might be able to use to enhance patient experiences in any number of ways. The work in this collection suggests there is more "scholarly activism" to be done, and that scholars in RHM are primed to apply their rhetorical savvy and literate practices in similar ways to advance advocacy on behalf of our patient participants and our own illness/patient communities.

Dying for a Feminist Healthcare Agenda

Dubriwny (2013) writes, "While public discourse about women's health issues points to the success of the women's health movement, the post-feminist nature of that discourse suggests the need to revisit what feminist health activism can look like—and accomplish—in the twenty-first century" (p. 145). Have feminists become complacent when it comes to our own healthcare? Have we accepted that equality in the doctor's office is when our PCP thinks our heart palpitations are anxiety? I don't think so. Feminist scholars in RHM can do as Dubriwny suggests in revisiting feminist healthcare activism, especially beyond the bikini— we can engage in healthcare activism for the whole woman's body.

This is especially important now, more than 20 years after Parrot and Condit, as we (the editors) developed this collection, and feminism itself is under attack. The first female presidential candidate ever to be elected by a major political party lost to man less than a month after the entire world heard tapes of him proudly saying, "You can do anything [to women]. Grab them by the pussy." Two years later, Trump's first Supreme Court candidate, Brett Kavanaugh, was confirmed, despite allegations that he sexually assaulted multiple women. Upon his confirmation, dozens of allegations against him of sexual misconduct were dismissed (Higgins, 2018). Now, with the Court leaning more conservatively, several states have banned abortion in various ways as they equip themselves to challenge *Roe v. Wade* (Stewart 2019).

The re-examination of *Roe v. Wade* is, however, only one constituent part of the larger Trump administration that could have serious effects on women's health. The ACA (or PPACA), signed into law during the Obama administration, makes it illegal for insurers to charge more for insurance to women just because they are women (gender rating); it also makes it illegal to deny coverage based on pre-existing conditions. The Trump administration has sought (at the time of this writing, unsuccessfully) to unravel the ACA, with specific attempts to undo parts of the bill that have been of most benefit to women. While reproductive rights, including access to birth control and safe abortions, are unequivocally necessary for both physical health and rhetorical embodiment, it is access to health insurance and healthcare despite pre-existing conditions that women need most if we are going to survive cardiac arrest.

In the US, we will not die from lack of access to birth control pills. But we will die from heart attacks, lung cancer, and Alzheimer's. Rhetoricians of health and medicine—especially those analyzing and enacting feminist rhetorics—can change this. Buchanan and Ryan (2010) offer a definition of "feminist rhetorics" as an "umbrella of sorts to encompass the many projects and purposes of ongoing work in the field" (p. xiii). While they list six projects and purposes, two are of particular relevance here: one purpose is "a theoretical mandate, namely exploring the shaping powers of language, gender ideology, and society; the location of subject(s) within these formations; and the ways these constructs inform the production, circulation, and interpretation of rhetorical texts"; another is "a practice, a scholarly endeavor capable of transforming the discipline of rhetoric through gender analysis, critique, and reformulation" (p. xiii). I see these purposes—a theoretical mandate and a transformative practice— manifested in the work collected in this volume.

Yet, Buchanan and Ryan (2010) describe another purpose of feminist rhetorics: "a political agenda directed toward promoting gender equity within the academy and society. In other words, the rhetorical work of this community of feminist teachers/scholars ... encourages others to think, believe, and act in ways that promote equal treatment and opportunities for women" (p. xiv). It is with this purpose, this project, that I believe we—rhetoricians in health and medicine— have work yet to do. As a co-editor of this collection, I am excited by the work that's included in this volume. Moreover, I believe I can speak for all of the contributors in this collection in saying that our next job is to take the work collected here, together with similar work collected elsewhere, and use it toward that action described by Buchanan and Ryan—in political agendas well beyond the academy; and take it to our hospitals, clinics, and laboratories; to our patient forums and online medical communities; to the pharmaceutical companies and health insurers; to lobbyists, congress, and the writers of health legislation; to our primary care doctors and our local clinics—to the places where rhetorical ingenuity can save our lives.

References

American Cancer Society. (2019a). "Breast cancer." Retrieved from www.cancer.org/cancer/breast-cancer/about/how-common-is-breast-cancer.html
American Cancer Society. (2019b). "Ovarian cancer." Retrieved from www.cancer.org/cancer/ovarian-cancer/causes-risks-prevention/prevention.html
Anand, S., Xie, C., Mehta, S., Franzosi, G., Joyner, C., Chrolavicius, S., Fox, K., & Yusuf, S. (2005). "Differences in the management and prognosis of women and men who suffer from acute coronary syndromes." *Journal of the American College of Cardiology*, 46(10), 1845–1851.
Arduser, L. (2017). *Living chronic: Agency and expertise in the rhetoric of diabetes.* Columbus, OH: Ohio State University Press.
Breast Cancer Action. (2019). "Priorities & theory of change." Retrieved from https://bcaction.org/about/priorities/
Buchanan, L., & Ryan, K. (2010). "Introduction: Walking and talking through the field of feminist rhetorics." In L. Buchanan & K. Ryan (Eds.). *Walking and talking feminist rhetorics: Landmark essays and controversies* (pp. xiii–xx). West Lafayette, IN: Parlor Press.
Centers for Disease Control. (2017). "Women and heart disease fact sheet." Retrieved from www.cdc.gov/dhdsp/data_statistics/fact_sheets/fs_women_heart.htm
Cushman, E. (1996). "The rhetorician as agent of social change." *College composition and communication*, 47(1), 7–28.
Dubriwny, T. (2013). *The vulnerable empowered woman: Feminism, postfeminism, and women's health.* New Brunswick, NJ: Rutgers University Press.
FORCE. (2019). "Health insurance appeals." Retrieved from www.facingourrisk.org/understanding-brca-and-hboc/information/finding-health-care/health-insurance-appeals/basics/how-to-file-appeal.php#text
Gulati, M. (2017). "Women and CV disease: Beyond the bikini." Retrieved from www.acc.org/latest-in-cardiology/articles/2017/05/15/15/women-and-cv-disease-beyond-the-bikini

Higgins, T. (2018). "Dozens of 'serious' conduct complaints against Justice Brett Kavanaugh are dismissed because he was confirmed to the Supreme Court." Retrieved from www.cnbc.com/2018/12/18/dozens-of-complaints-against-brett-kavanaugh-dismissed.html

Lichtman, J., Leifheit, E., Safdar, B., Bao, H., Krumholz, H., Lorenze, N., Daneshvar, M., Spertus, J., & D'Onofrio, G. (2018). "Sex differences in the presentation and perception of symptoms among young patients with myocardial infarction." *Circulation*, 137, 781–790.

National Football League Communications. (2015). "NFL supports national breast cancer awareness month with a crucial catch campaign." Retrieved from https://nflcommunications.com/Pages/NFL-Supports-National-Breast-Cancer-Awareness-Month-With-A-Crucial-Catch-Campaign.aspx

North American Menopause Society (2018). "New study demonstrates increased risk of heart disease after hysterectomy." Retrieved from www.eurekalert.org/pub_releases/2018-01/tnam-nsd010318.php

Parrot, R.L., & Condit, C.M. (1996). "Introduction: Priorities and agendas in communicating about women's reproductive health." In R.L. Parrot & C.M. Condit (Eds.). *Evaluating women's health messages: A resource book* (pp. 1–12). Thousand Oaks, CA: Sage.

Parthasarathy, S. (2014). "Awash in pink, but breast cancer awareness isn't a cure." Retrieved from https://theconversation.com/awash-in-pink-but-breast-cancer-awareness-isnt-a-cure-31758

Sartor, A. (2015). "What the frack? Drill rig goes pink(washing) for breast cancer." Retrieved from https://bcaction.org/2012/11/15/what-the-frack-drill-rig-goes-pinkwashing-for-breast-cancer/

Scott, J.B., & Melançon, L. (2018). "Manifesting methodologies for the rhetoric of health & medicine." In L. Melançon & J.B. Scott (Eds.). *Methodologies for the rhetoric of health and medicine* (pp. 1–23). New York: Routledge.

Spatz, E., Curry, L., Masoudi, F., Zhou, S., Strait, K., Gross, C., Curtis, J., … & Krumholz, H. (2015). "The variation in recovery: Role of gender on outcomes of young AMI patients (VIRGO) classification system: A taxonomy for young women with acute myocardial infarction." *Circulation*, 132, 1710–1718.

Stewart, S. F. (2019). "Amid wave of states restricting abortion, advocates step up efforts to get women to clinics." Retrieved from www.centerforhealthjournalism.org/2019/05/28/amid-wave-states-restricting-abortion-advocates-get-women-clinics?fbclid=IwAR2hqMNS5l31rTvW5UzyymHLiX9hc54f5IcWA69Djt5Yu-YktfvVtxH2aSk

Yong, E. (2018). "Women more likely to survive heart attacks if treated by female doctors." Retrieved from www.theatlantic.com/science/archive/2018/08/women-more-likely-to-survive-heart-attacks-if-treated-by-female-doctors/566837/

Women's Brain Health Initiative. (2015). "Sex differences in research prove more valuable than ever before." Retrieved from https://womensbrainhealth.org/think-twice/beyond-the-bikini

CONTRIBUTORS

About the Editors

Jamie White-Farnham is Associate Professor and Writing Coordinator at the University of Wisconsin-Superior, where she teaches first-year writing and courses in the writing major. Her research is focused on writing and rhetoric that influences the lives and material conditions of women, and her work has appeared in *Rhetoric Review*, *Community Literacy Journal*, and *College English*.

Bryna Siegel Finer is Associate Professor and Director of Writing Across the Curriculum at Indiana University of Pennsylvania. Some of her scholarly work can be found in *Rhetoric Review*, *Teaching English in the Two-Year College*, *Praxis*, and the *Journal of Teaching Writing*. With Jamie White-Farnham, she is the co-editor of *Writing Program Architecture: Thirty Cases for Reference and Research*, published by Utah State University Press in November 2017.

Cathryn Molloy is Associate Professor in James Madison University's School of Writing, Rhetoric and Technical Communication, where she serves as Director of Undergraduate Studies and teaches in the undergraduate and graduate programs. An assistant editor for the journal *Rhetoric of Health and Medicine*, her work focuses on issues of credibility in health contexts. Her research has appeared in *Rhetoric Society Quarterly*, *Qualitative Inquiry*, and *Rhetoric Review*.

About the Contributors

Kristin Marie Bivens is Associate Professor of English at Harold Washington College. She is an associate editor for the Foundations and Innovations in Technical and Professional Communication book series and a 2018–2019 Newberry Library Scholar-in-Residence. Her research interests include communication/ rhetoric in acute care, activist, and political contexts. Her work appears in the *Journal of Communication Inquiry, Health Communication, Communication Design Quarterly,* and the *Journal of Business and Technical Communication.* Her website is www.kristinbivens.com.

April Cabral is a wife and mother of two from Somerset, MA, who is currently living with metastatic breast cancer. Since her cancer diagnosis three years ago, she has worked tirelessly to raise awareness and funds for Metastatic Breast Cancer Research at Dana Farber Cancer Institute through the Jimmy Fund.

Kirsti Cole is a Professor of Composition, Rhetoric, and Literature at Minnesota State University. She is the faculty chair of the Teaching Writing Graduate Certificate and the MS in Communication and Composition. Her work appears in the *Journal of Communication Inquiry, Feminist Media Studies, College English,* and *Harlot,* and she has a number of chapters in collections focused on communication, composition, and feminist studies. She is the editor of *Feminist Challenges or Feminist Rhetorics?* (2014) and the co-editor of *Surviving Sexism in Academia* (2017).

Marleah Dean (Ph.D., Texas A&M University) is an Assistant Professor at the University of South Florida. Her research investigates how patients, families, and healthcare providers exchange information, manage uncertainty, and make decisions regarding issues of hereditary cancer. Her work has been published in journals such as *Academic Medicine, Patient Education & Counseling, Qualitative Health Research, Health Communication, Journal of Health Communication,* and *Journal of Genetic Counseling.* Her website is www.cancercommunicationresearch.com.

Lori Beth De Hertogh is an Assistant Professor in the School of Writing, Rhetoric and Technical Communication at James Madison University, where she teaches courses in feminist rhetorics, rhetorics of health and medicine, digital rhetorics, and more. Her work has appeared in *Computers and Composition, Journal of Business and Technical Communication, Enculturation, Composition Studies,* and *Ada: A Journal of Gender, New Media, & Technology.* Her website is www.loribethdehertogh.com.

Lisa DeTora, Associate Professor and Director of STEM Writing at Hofstra University, teaches scientific writing, metacognition, narrative medicine, disability studies and composition. She also serves as guest faculty in medical humanities at the Donald and Barbara Zucker School of Medicine at Hofstra/Northwell. Her recent publications have appeared in *Communication Design Quarterly, Rhetoric of Health and Medicine, Current Medical Research and Opinion,* and *The International Journal of Clinical Practice.*

Erin Fitzgerald is a Ph.D. candidate and Editorial Assistant of the peer-reviewed journal, *Written Communication*, at Auburn University. Her research focuses on rhetoric, genre uptake, feminist theory, ethics of care, public policy, and circulation of health and medicine discourse to specific stakeholder groups. She has presented her work at the Feminisms and Rhetorics Conference, the Southwest Popular American Culture Association Annual Conference, and the Conference on College Composition and Communication (CCCC). Her work has appeared in *Kairos: A Journal of Rhetoric, Technology, and Pedagogy*.

Oriana Gilson is a Ph.D. candidate in the English Studies Department at Illinois State University, specializing in rhetoric, composition, and technical and professional communication. Her research interests include rhetorics of efficiency within public policy, rhetorics of health and medicine, and usability. She is the Assistant Editor for *Rhetoric Review*.

Kim Hensley Owens is Associate Professor of English and Director of the University Writing Program at Northern Arizona University. Her scholarship focuses on rhetorical agency, embodied rhetorics, and pedagogy. Recent publications include articles in *College English* and *Present Tense* and her Southern Illinois University Press book, *Writing Childbirth: Women's Rhetorical Agency in Labor and Online* (2015).

Janna Klostermann is a Ph.D. candidate in Carleton University's Department of Sociology and Anthropology. Her academic and artistic work reveals social and historical conditions of care through the work and words of care providers and activists. Her work has recently appeared in *Ethnography and Education*, *Literacy and Numeracy Studies*, and *Women Studies Quarterly*.

Amy Koerber is Professor in Communication Studies and Associate Dean for Faculty Success & Inclusion in the College of Media & Communication at Texas Tech University. Research interests include health and science communication, with a specific focus on women's health issues. Her most recent book, *From Hysteria to Hormones: A Rhetorical History*, was published by Penn State University Press in April 2018.

Donna Laux earned an M.A. in English from the University of Wisconsin-Milwaukee, and is now semiretired. Much of her career was focused on women's health. She was the Founding Director of the Center for Endometriosis Care (CEC) in Atlanta, and is currently an admin for Nancy's Nook, a Facebook group for people with endometriosis that has more than 53,000 members worldwide.

Jennifer Malkowski is an Assistant Professor of Communication Arts and Sciences at California State University, Chico. Her research and teaching interests lie at the intersections of public health communication, medical professionalism, and biotechnological controversy. Her work has appeared in *Health Communication* and the *Journal of Medical Humanities*. She is co-editor of a forthcoming (2019) special issue of *Rhetoric of Health and Medicine* focused on Rhetoric of Public Health.

Marissa McKinley is Assistant Teaching Professor of English at Quinnipiac University. Her research interests include the rhetoric of health and medicine, feminist theory and pedagogy, and writing program administration. Marissa's scholarship has been presented at the Conference on College Composition and Communication, Feminisms and Rhetoric, and at the Rhetoric Society of America. In addition, Marissa's work has been featured in *Across the Disciplines* and the *WAC-GO Newsletter*.

Laurie McMillan is Associate Professor of English and Chair of the English and Modern Language Studies Department at Pace University. Her research focuses on feminist writing and rhetoric as well as composition studies. She published a composition textbook, *Focus on Writing: What College Students Want to Know* (Broadview Press, 2019), and is working on a book manuscript entitled *Slut Rhetoric: Social Media, Pop Culture, and Politics*.

Maria Novotny is an Assistant Professor of English at the University of Wisconsin-Oshkosh, where she teaches courses in writing and rhetoric. Her research oscillates around the intersections of community literacy, health activism, and cultural rhetorics. The focus of this work centers on her collaboration with "The ART of Infertility," a traveling arts exhibit portraying representations of reproductive loss for educational and advocacy purposes. Her work has appeared in *Computers and Composition*, *Harlot*, *Peitho*, and *Reflections*.

Cynthia Pengilly (Ph.D., Old Dominion University) is an Assistant Professor of English and Co-Director of the Technical Writing Program at Central Washington University. She teaches courses in composition, technical, and professional communication, visual rhetoric, and cultural studies. Her research is focused on the rhetoric and culture of technology and explores the implications of (mostly online) technologies on everyday, lived experiences, such as women's health and pedagogical identity. She has several forthcoming articles and book chapters.

Janeen Qadri is a Lupus warrior; she advocates for the Lupus community by providing educational blogs on managing Lupus through integrative medicine. She serves as a board member of Lupus Alliance of Upstate New York.

Sheri Rysdam is Associate Professor in Literacies & Composition at Utah Valley University. Her scholarship in feminist medical rhetorics is inspired in part by her work as a volunteer doula. She also publishes on responding to student writing and rhetorics of political economy. Her work appears in journals and edited collections such as *Peer Pressure, Peer Power: Collaborative Peer Review and Response in the Writing Classroom*, the *Journal for Expanded Perspectives on Learning*, and *Issues in Writing*.

Billie R. Tadros is an Assistant Professor in the Department of English & Theatre at the University of Scranton, where she teaches courses in poetry and poetry writing. Her research interests concern women's embodiment; narratives of illness, injury, and disability; and constructions and representations of mental illness and suicide. She is the author of two books of poems: *The Tree We Planted and Buried You In*, published by Otis Books in 2018, and *Was Body*, forthcoming from Indolent Books.

Ann E. Wallace is an Associate Professor of English at New Jersey City University. As a composition specialist focused on illness literature and trauma, she has written on the intersections of the fields in *Intima: A Journal of Narrative Medicine* and *Transformations: The Journal of Inclusive Scholarship and Pedagogy*. She also explores her experiences with ovarian cancer and multiple sclerosis through poetry and prose, and her collection *Counting by Sevens* was published by Main Street Rag Publishing in 2019.

Kelly A. Whitney is an Assistant Professor of English and Coordinator of the Professional Writing Minor at The Ohio State University at Mansfield. Her research and teaching focus on ethics and materiality in medical and technical writing.

INDEX

Note: Page numbers in *italics* refer to figures.

religious rights arguments 194;
slut-shaming narratives and reproductive
rights 192–194; three responses to
Limbaugh 191–192, 196–200; women
of color and poor women 193
research, advocacy through 158, 159
RESOLVE 66, 69
Restaino, J. 178
restitution narrative 126
rhetoric of doubt 48, 49, 50
rhetorical autoethnography 14–24; diary
entries 15, 16, 17–19; forms of advocacy
20, 22; hip labral tear blog posts 20–22;
private breast lump biopsies essay 15–16;
providing relief from trauma 16; for
psychological benefit 21; public speech on
medical insurance cover 16–17; a snapshot
of thinking at a particular time 22–23;
wrist issue diary entries 17–19; writing a
seminar paper on writing in pain 19–20
rhetorical deterrent model, medical
discourse acting as 47–50
rhetorical ingenuity, defining 2–3;
demonstrations and practices of 26, 32,
35, 38, 42, 79, 84–86, 150, 174, 187; as
microactivism 21, 23; sites of 112; agents
of 115, 117–119; challenges of 165
rhetorical listening 95
rhetorics of efficiency 138, 139–140; as a
framework for analyzing breastfeeding
policy and discourse 140–144
rhythm method 170–171, *171*
rhetorics/rhetoricians in/of health and
medicine (RHM), as activists/ism 4, 209;
epistemologies and theories of 6, 103,
111; research in/by 3, 6–7; and women's
health 2, 46, 204, 207; goals for/calls to
7, 56, 119, 145, 205, 210–211
Rich, A. 91, 100, 179
Roe v. Wade 210
Royne, M.B. 34, 35, 41
Rudd, A. 183
Ryan, K. 210, 211

Saldaña, J. 37
Santorum, R. 192
scavenging 180, 182–183
scholarly activism 207, 209
Scott, J.B. 7, 15, 79, 111, 112, 113,
177, 207
Sedgwick, E.K. 26, 27, 28
Segal, J.Z. 4, 6, 15, 26, 27, 28, 31, 38, 94,
178, 179

Seigel, M. 91–92, 109
self-action, PCOS and taking 40–41, 42
self-disclosure of infertility: and health
activism 60, 63–66, 68–69; risks of
69–70
self-empowerment: through online
reference and support groups 36, 45; *see
also* patient empowerment
self-research, myPCOSteam and 40–41, 42
Selzer, J. 178, 179
Setoyama, Y. 42
Seymour, W. 125
Shainman, A.B. 156–157
sharing experiences, advocacy through
154–157; *see also* knowledge sharing,
patient-to-patient
Shildrick, M. 77–78
Sims, J.M. 81–82
Sinor, J. 15, 17, 23
slut-shaming *see* reproductive rights and
responses to slut shaming
social imaginaries 177; women's voices
altering AIDS' 182–184
Sontag, S. 27
speculum 81–82
Steuber, K.R. 70
stories: and counterstories of infertility
64–66, 70; infant feeding 145; outside
academia shared in online spaces 145;
sharing birth 93, 98–100; women
runners sharing 129–130
Stormer, N. 79
storying 180
strategic contemplation 95, 96–97
survivor in illness discourse, metaphor of
28–29

Tarzian, A.J. 127
Taylor, D. 180, 181, 183, 184, 185,
186, 187
Tesch, R. 37
tetanus vaccine 116
textual agency 122, 124, 127, 128
"Third Time's a Charm" campaign 103,
106–107
Trump administration 210

UNICEF 137, 138
Uthappa, N.R. 63

vaccination: contested terrain of 111;
discourses 103–104, 111–112, 112–113,
118–119; early programs 112; "herd

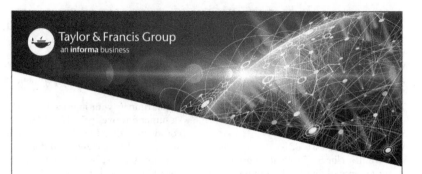